Psychoneuroendocrinology c
Sport and Exercise

Psychoneuroendocrinology is the study of the interaction between hormones, the brain and human behaviour. This is the first book to examine psychoneuroendocrinology in the context of sport and exercise, offering a comprehensive review of current research and assessment techniques and highlighting directions for future research.

The book explores the bidirectional links between hormones and behaviour, and draws important conclusions for how their study will aid in understanding the bidirectional link between sport and behaviour that is central to the psychology of sport and exercise. It presents the key hormones that underpin behaviour in a sporting context, including the description of their physiologic mechanisms and behavioural effects. The book reports benchmark standards for the assessment and analysis of hormonal influences of behaviour in sport, and examines practical issues and contexts such as emotional state (anxiety, for example), overtraining and stress.

Psychoneuroendocrinology of Sport and Exercise is a breakthrough text that will be of interest to all advanced students and researchers working in the psychology and physiology of sport and exercise.

Felix Ehrlenspiel is lecturer at TU München and received his PhD in Psychology in 2006 from the University of Potsdam. His research is concerned with behavioural, psychological and neuroendocrine responses to competitions, and he currently teaches athletes and students how to deal with these responses.

Katharina Strahler M.Sc., works as a clinical psychologist for children and adolescents. She is currently completing her PhD at the Technische Universität München, Germany. Her research interests are psychoneuroendocrinology of stress in sport, competitive anxiety and doping prevention interventions.

Routledge Research in Sport and Exercise Science

The *Routledge Research in Sport and Exercise Science* series is a showcase for cutting-edge research from across the sport and exercise sciences, including physiology, psychology, biomechanics, motor control, physical activity and health, and every core sub-discipline. Featuring the work of established and emerging scientists and practitioners from around the world, and covering the theoretical, investigative and applied dimensions of sport and exercise, this series is an important channel for new and groundbreaking research in the human movement sciences.

Also available in this series:

Psychoneuroendocrinology of Sport and Exercise

Foundations, markers, trends

**Edited by Felix Ehrlenspiel and
Katharina Strahler**

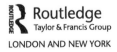

Routledge
Taylor & Francis Group

LONDON AND NEW YORK

First published 2012
by Routledge
2 Park Square, Milton Park, Abingdon, Oxfordshire OX14 4RN

Simultaneously published in the USA and Canada
by Routledge
711 Third Avenue, New York, NY 10017

First issued in paperback 2014

Routledge is an imprint of the Taylor & Francis Group, an informa business

British Library Cataloguing in Publication Data
A catalogue record for this book is available from the British Library

Library of Congress Cataloging in Publication Data
  Psychoneuroendocrinology of sport and exercise : foundations,
  markers, trends / edited by Felix Ehrlenspiel and Katharina Strahler.
    p. cm.—(Routledge research in sport and exercise science)
  1. Sports. 2. Exercise. 3. Psychoneuroendocrinology.
  I. Ehrlenspiel, Felix. II. Strahler, Katharina.
  RC1235.P79 2012
  613.7′1—dc23
  2011039989

ISBN: 978–0–415–67834–6 (hbk)
ISBN: 978-1-138-79576-1 (pbk)

Typeset in Goudy
by Swales & Willis Ltd, Exeter, Devon

To Lena and Lisabeth, Marcus and Joshua

Contents

PART III
Research trends   139
KATHARINA STRAHLER AND FELIX EHRLENSPIEL

Contributors

Henning Budde, Reykjavik University, School of Science and Engineering, Department of Sport Science and Physical Education, Menntavegi 1, Nauthólsvík, 101 Reykjavík, Iceland. Email: henning.budde@gmx.net

Felix Ehrlenspiel, Technische Universität München, Lehrstuhl für Sportpsychologie, Uptown München – Campus D, Georg-Brauchle-Ring 60/62, 80992 München, Germany. Email: felix.ehrlenspiel@tum.de

Edith Filaire, Université d' Orléans, UFR STAPS, 2 allée du Château, F-45062 Orléans Cedex 2, France. Email: edith.filaire@univ-orleans.fr

Elisabeth Klumbies, Technische Universität Dresden, Professur Biopsychologie, Zellescher Weg 19, D-01069 Dresden, Germany. Email: klumbies@biopsych.tu-dresden.de

Ulrike Rimmele, New York University, Psychology Department, 6 Washington Place, New York, NY 10003, USA. Email: ur228@nyu.edu

Alicia Salvador, Universitat de València, Avinguda Blasco Ibanyez 21, E-46010 València, Spain. Email: Alicia.Salvador@uv.es

Martin Schönfelder, Technische Universität München, Lehrstuhl für Sport und Gesundheitsförderung, Uptown München – Campus D, Georg-Brauchle-Ring 60/62, 80992 München, Germany. Email: martin.schoenfelder@tum.de

Thorsten Schulz, Technische Universität München, Lehrstuhl für Sport und Gesundheitsförderung, Uptown München – Campus D, Georg-Brauchle-Ring 60/62, 80992 München, Germany. Email: thorsten.schulz@tum.de

Silvan Steiner, Universität Bern, Institut für Sportwissenschaft, Alpeneggstrasse 22, CH-3012 Bern, Switzerland. Email: silvan.steiner@ispw.unibe.ch

Jana Strahler, Philipps-Universität Marburg, Lichtenberg-Professor für Klinische Biopsychologie, Gutenbergstrasse 18, 35032 Marburg, Germany. Email: strahler@uni-marburg.de

Katharina Strahler, AMEOS Klinikum Ueckermünde, Klinik für Kinder- und Jugendpsychiatrie, Psychosomatik und Psychotherapie, Ravensteinstraße 23, D-17373 Ueckermünde, Germany. Email: kstr.kjp@ueckermuende.ameos.de

Ferran Suay, Universitat de València, Departament de Psicobiologia, Avinguda Blasco Ibanyez 21, E-46010 València, Spain. Email: suay@valencia.edu

Mirko Wegner, Humboldt-Universität zu Berlin, Institut für Sportwissenschaft, Abteilung Sportpsychologie, Philippstraße 13, D-10115 Berlin, Germany. Email: mirko.wegner@cms.hu-berlin.de

Claudia Windisch, Jacobs Center on Lifelong Learning – JCLL, Jacobs University Bremen GmbH, Campus Ring 1, D-28759 Bremen, Germany. Email: c.windisch@jacobs-university.de

Preface

The most exciting phrase to hear in science, the one that heralds new discoveries, is not 'Eureka!' but 'That's funny'.

(Isaac Asimov)

The idea of this book developed from the observation that there was growing interest in psychoneuroendocrinological research within sport psychology, and that researchers genuinely associated in psychoneuroendocrinology were becoming interested in sport as a test bed for their theories. But when we started doing research of our own, we found it funny to discover that a comprehensive introduction specific to our field was missing. We are greatly indebted to Routledge, specifically Simon Whitmore and Joshua Wells, for supporting us in our endeavour to fill this void. Despite the scepticism of some early reviewers, they believed that some of the contributors, most of them not yet fully established and visible, would still have the expertise necessary for the success of this project. Possibly underlining the observation that psychoneuroendocrinology of sport and exercise is still emerging as a field of sports science is not only the age and experience of the contributors, but also the fact that five children were born to them during the writing of the book! We hope that, much like our babies, interest in psychoneuroendocrinology in sport and exercise continues to grow within research.

Acknowledgements

Support for this book project was provided in part from the German Federal Institute of Sports Science that assisted us in the early stages (BISp AZ 07100108–09). Nils Bühring, Andrea Geipel, Franziska Lefrank, Tom Kossak and Eva Zier provided invaluable help with editing, correcting and proofreading the manuscript, Ed Beese also helped with correcting early versions. We would also like to thank Professor Jürgen Beckmann for providing important resources, a stimulating discussion at the staff retreat and for silently accepting the time that went into this project. Less silent was each one of our two newborn children. We thus thank our spouses Lena and Marcus, respectively, for their extra hours of cradling, feeding and lulling to bed and for their continuous support.

We are grateful to the following experts in the field who were willing to review chapters of the book and whose comments greatly enhanced each chapter: Dr Justin M. Carré, Duke University, Dr Aaron Coutts, University of Technology, Sydney, Dr Daniel Erlacher, Universität Bern, Dr Markus Gerber, Universität Basel and Dr Joanne Thatcher, Aberystwyth University.

Part I

Foundations of a psychoneuroendocrinology of sport and exercise

Katharina Strahler and Felix Ehrlenspiel

In this first section the editors, Felix Ehrlenspiel and Katharina Strahler, lay the ground for a psychoneuroendocrinology of sport and exercise by first showing that the psychology of sport and exercise encompasses various perspectives and orientations. After introducing psychoneuroendocrinology, a model is described that might aid in the use of psychoneuroendocrinology for the integration of these perspectives and orientations. In the second chapter of this section, Jana Strahler and Elisabeth Klumbies lay the foundation for the understanding of the following sections. They describe the physiological basics of psychoneuroendocrinology, how studies in psychoneuroendocrinology are designed and how the various markers may be assessed and analysed.

1 Introduction

Felix Ehrlenspiel and Katharina Strahler

One of the fascinating aspects of practising sports or engaging in physical exercise is that we can immediately experience 'psychology'. We engage in social interaction with our sports team members or our exercise group, and we feel how this interaction affects how we perform as a team or how motivated we are to go and exercise again next week. We experience how each successful basketball free throw or how each extra weight lifted leads to greater self-confidence and a good feeling, but we also experience how worries or a lack of concentration lead to performance failure, or how a lack of motivation keeps us from exercising more often. We also perceive general well-being and our good health after a game of football or exercise session but we also feel the rising tension in our body before the competition or the knot in the stomach when our neighbour again outlasts us on the treadmill.

These phenomena are not just exciting to the individual engaged in sport activities, they are also the subject of scientific study. In sport psychology, the study of human behaviour and experience in sport is aimed at understanding and predicting behaviour but also at eventually applying knowledge gained from this study (see Gill, 2000; Weinberg and Gould, 2003). Recent developments in the field of sport psychology have yielded an increasing interest in the biological basis of phenomenal experiences. Although within this area the brain itself is at the centre of study, there is growing interest in the role of hormones in how the brain exerts its behavioural control – and in how behaviour affects the brain. Before describing a framework for the study of the role of hormones in sport behaviour, we first describe in more detail how human behaviour and experience in sport are studied.

Sport psychology

The scientific study of the 'psychology' experience in sport is thus concerned with human behaviour and experience in this context (see Gill, 2000; Weinberg and Gould, 2003). Here and throughout the book 'sport' is used in a more generic fashion. Following the European usage, we understand sport as 'all forms of physical activity which, through casual or organized participation, aim at expressing or improving physical fitness and mental well-being, forming social relationships or obtaining results in competition at all levels' (European Sports Charter: Council of Europe, 2001). In the Anglo- and especially American usage, sport is usually associated with the aim of obtaining results in competition but not the other goals – which are referred to as exercise – thus representing a narrower meaning. Consequently, the use of sport psychology to describe the field has been considered too narrow, and the term 'sport and exercise psychology' has been established (see Gill, 2000). In this chapter as well as throughout the book, the term sport psychology and sport will be used to describe both sport and exercise. Whenever it is necessary to distinguish the two explicitly, the precise term will be used. As the definition of the European Council also shows, physical activity is an even more generic term, including activities such as climbing a staircase, running to catch the bus or cleaning your room. Those will not be the focus of this book.

The term sport psychology incorporates two disciplines of study and research: sport science and psychology. But there is some discussion as to whether sport psychology should be considered a subdiscipline of sport science (e.g. Gill, 2000) or whether sport psychology is actually derived from psychology (Anshel, 2003). In her assignment of sport psychology to sport science, Gill argues that sport psychology lies in the middle of a physical-to-social continuum with ties to all other areas of sport science. What makes sport psychology a subdiscipline of sport science is that it integrates theories and information from the other sport science fields and psychology to create unique knowledge specific to the field of sport (Gill, 2000). Anshel (2003), however, argues that sport psychology is derived from the traditional disciplines of psychology such as social psychology, developmental psychology or cognitive psychology. Nevertheless, the development of sport psychology as a field of study and research is rooted in physical education (Anshel, 2003). Thus most sport psychology programmes at university level are located in sport science departments (often under the name of kinesiology or human movement) rather than in psychology departments (Morris *et al.*, 2003).

Although the discussion whether sport psychology is a subdiscipline of sport science or of psychology may seem a bit academic, it clearly shows that study and research can address behaviour and experience in sport from either of the two perspectives by laying an emphasis either on psychology or on sport (Weinberg and Gould, 2003, in similar vein use the term 'objective'). The first perspective, which one might call the *psychology perspective*, views the field from psychology and is concerned with the effects of 'the mind', that is, psychological states or variables on sport behaviour. This perspective is probably the most common view taken by research in sport psychology, and it is also the oldest. The earliest studies in sport psychology, carried out at the end of the nineteenth century, found that performance in a motor skill was enhanced in the presence of others (Triplett, 1898). And the classic study by Yerkes and Dodson (1908), although originally investigating the behaviour of rats, led to the investigation of the effects of arousal and anxiety on the performance of sports tasks. This line of research also shows the complexity of the relation between psychology and sport: the relation between arousal, anxiety and sports performance is still being investigated today (cf. reviews by Craft *et al.*, 2003; Woodman and Hardy, 2003) and it appears that not only do more mental and more physical components need to be separated but also the relationship appears to be highly individual (Hanin, 2000).

The second perspective, which one might call the *sport perspective*, views the field from within sport and is concerned with the effects of sport behaviour on the mind. The key question here is whether and how sports activities affect mental well-being and health. With reference to the roman proverb '*mens sana in corpore sano*' it is generally assumed that sport, but especially physical exercise, has positive effects on mood and affect but also reactivity to stress (e.g. Gerber, 2008; Wipfli *et al.*, 2008).

Independent of the perspective of sport psychology, within research, but also within practice or application, three main orientations may be distinguished (Weinberg and Gould, 2003). The *social–psychological orientation* is interested in the interaction in the sports context of an individual with his or her environment, especially with other individuals; it is also interested in how our assumptions about the world form our cognitions, decisions and behaviour. With respect to the psychology perspective, for example, teams have been found to perform better if they exhibit at least some task cohesion (Carron *et al.*, 2002), and exercising in a group generally leads to a better adherence to an exercise programme (Burke *et al.*, 2008). With respect to the sport perspective it has been shown that, for example, motor experience in a sport activity influences referees' perceptual decisions (Dosseville *et al.*, 2011).

The second main orientation may be labelled the *cognitive–behavioural orientation*, as it is interested not only in the role of cognitions in the determination of behaviour, such as thoughts and feelings, but also attentional or motivational processes. Again, from a psychology perspective research has found, for example, that anxiety associated with evaluative situations in sport leads to a more controlled movement execution and consequently performance failure (Beilock and Carr, 2001; Ehrlenspiel *et al.*, 2010) and that focusing on the platform rather than on the feet enhances motor learning in a balancing task in older adults (Chiviakowsky *et al.*, 2010). From a sport perspective it has been found that athletes learn to develop self-regulatory skills (Szymanski *et al.*, 2004) and that physical exercise has been shown to lead to improved cognitive functioning even in elderly persons (Erickson and Kramer, 2009).

The third orientation identified by Weinberg and Gould (2003) is interested in the physiological processes underlying or accompanying behaviour and psychological states in sport. Again, from a psychology perspective research has shown, for example, that the ability to regulate physiological responses such as skin conductance or muscle tone can lead to better sport performance (Bar-Eli and Blumenstein, 2004). And from a sport perspective, winning a competition in a fight sport is thought to lead to increased levels of testosterone (Filaire *et al.*, 2001), commonly associated with a higher level of aggression, and acute exercise has been linked with increased alpha-band activity in the EEG (e.g. Crabbe and Dishman, 2004), commonly associated with a relaxed state.

Although the social–psychological and cognitive–behavioural orientations are still dominant, the psychophysiological orientation has more recently received increased attention in sport and exercise psychology research. This is evidenced, for example, by the publication of a review textbook entitled *Psychobiology of Physical Activity*, edited by Acevedo and Ekkekakis (2006a). This discusses the contribution that psychobiology has made to our understanding of all questions in the field of sport psychology, and gives examples concerning the psychobiology of physical activity and cognition, emotion, mental health and human performance. Understanding psychobiology as the broader term, the volume encompasses methods from psychophysiology (for example measuring cortical activity or skin conductance), physiology (heart rate) and also neurophysiology (assessment of neurotransmitters), psychoneuroimmunology and psychoneuroendocrinology (assessment of cytokines or hormones).

Acevedo and Ekkekakis (2006b) also chart the progress of the study of sport and exercise psychology from a psychobiological orientation following earlier and less positive assessments by Hatfield and Landers (1983) or Dishman (1994). They also clearly point to the need for an integrative science that respects the multiple levels of analysis of human behaviour in sport (for example the social, cognitive and physiological orientations). The social–psychological and cognitive–behavioural orientations have long demonstrated a neglect of the psychobiological orientation, as evidenced, for example, by a lack of this orientation in current textbooks of sport psychology (cf. Gill, 2000; Anshel, 2003; Weinberg and Gould, 2003).

It appears that the progress of psychobiology within sport psychology has also been hindered by a neglect of the psychological or cognitive orientation. Acevedo and Ekkekakis (2006b) argue that for progress of sport and exercise psychology to occur it is important to seek evidence from these different levels of analysis and to relate each level or orientation to one another. Not only must psychological theories be physiologically plausible (and testable), but psychobiological study must also be based on sound psychological theories. Importantly, this integration of the orientations needs to occur within sport psychology, because theories and models of behaviour and experience *in sport* are integrated into biological theories. Consequently, this integration also needs to be pursued by *sport psychologists*, because they have the knowledge of the psychological phenomena, questions, theories and models in sport. However, for this integration to occur within sport psychology by sport psychologists, a better understanding of psychobiological theories and methods is necessary.

To a large extent, psychobiology in sport and exercise psychology today is concerned with neuroscience with a focus on electrophysiological and brain imaging studies. In this book we want to provide insights into an exciting field of psychobiology that should receive more attention and that should complement the current trend of neurophysiology in sport because it allows a better understanding of the interaction between the brain and the body: this is the field of psychoneuroendocrinology.

Psychoneuroendocrinology

As the term implies, the basis of psychoneuroendocrinology is the study of the interaction and the interdependence of psychological, neurological and endocrine mechanisms (e.g. McCubbin, 2000). It is based on *behavioural endocrinology*, which shows how the endocrine system affects behaviour and vice versa. Furthermore, it not only acknowledges the role of the central nervous system (CNS) in mediating these relations between the endocrine system and behaviour but it also expands the level of analysis by including psychological variables (i.e. the mind – e.g. mental and affective states) as effects and causes of the activity of the endocrine system.

The endocrine system and behaviour

The endocrine system regulates, integrates and controls the bodily functions of an organism (Nelson, 2005) and thus serves a function very similar to that of the nervous system: it signals information. The information within the endocrine system is communicated through chemical substances called hormones that are secreted – mostly into the bloodstream – by various endocrine glands throughout the body. The name derives from the Greek words *endo*, meaning 'inside or within' and *crinis*, meaning 'secrete'.

Hormones attach to target tissue or organs possibly far from the gland and exert effects on the functioning of this tissue. This interaction between hormone and target tissue is very specific: to exert its effect, a hormone needs to be able to bind to a specific receptor. Thus, whether and how much effect a hormone exerts depends both on the hormone (e.g. its concentration in the blood) and on its receptors (e.g. their location or number). By regulating, integrating and controlling bodily functions, the endocrine system coordinates physiology and behaviour (Becker and Breedlove, 2002).

The field of endocrinology is today traced back to an experiment by German physician and physiologist Arnold Berthold (Nelson, 2005). He observed the development and behaviour of roosters that had been castrated as cockerels and that either had their testes completely removed, had their testes reimplanted or had testes transplanted from another cockerel. While the cockerels with reimplanted or transplanted testes eventually showed normal development into a rooster with typical behaviour such as crowing or engaging in aggressive and sexual behaviour, the cockerels with completely removed testes developed into capons, they did not crow and showed no signs of mating behaviour. This experiment demonstrated that behaviour could be under non-neural control – the transplanted testes functioned after all nerves were severed. It demonstrated that the testes produced some kind of substance that circulated in the blood and had specific effects on development and behaviour. The substance, a hormone, is now known as testosterone.

Later studies have proven that testosterone plays a major role in the development of sexual differentiation and controlling masculine sexual behaviour. In fact, the hormonal control of sexual behaviour, or more general, reproductive behaviour, is a prime example of hormonal behaviour control and also a prime concern of behavioural endocrinology. Other main functions of hormones are the coordination of growth and development, social behaviours such as aggression, cooperation or parenting and maintaining homeostasis.

Reproductive behaviour is also a good example of the integrative and coordinative function of the endocrine system, because both physiology and behaviour are integrated and coordinated to produce an effect. For example, testosterone leads to both the production of sperm in the testes and increases the likelihood of mating behaviour. This is important because only through mating behaviour can sperm be disseminated, and only because of sperm production is mating behaviour effective. A similar coordinative function can be observed in the metabolic system: before awakening in the morning, several hormones (e.g. cortisol) are secreted in anticipation of the activity of the upcoming day in order to provide energy through elevated levels of blood glucose.

Beyond the control of behaviour and the coordination with physiology, hormones also play an important part in the regulation of the internal environment. Homeostasis is the term coined by Walter B Cannon (1929) for the process organisms use to maintain a relatively stable or constant internal milieu. Systems that are maintained in homeostasis include the fluid system, energy balance or body temperature, but organisms also seek to maintain optimal blood concentrations of various constituents such as glucose, proteins or electrolytes. Maintaining homeostasis again involves the coordination of physiology and behaviour and the integration of various hormones. For example, eating food leads to the supply of metabolic fuels such as glucose or fatty acids. But these fuels can only be stored for further energy expenditure (anabolism) if the hormone insulin is present. If energy is needed, for example during strenuous exercise, hormones are needed not only to release the energy (catabolism) but also to prevent anabolism via insulin.

Neural interaction with the endocrine system

There is a close reciprocal relation between the endocrine system and the nervous system. The primary interface between the two systems is the hypothalamus and it can be considered the neural control centre of the endocrine system. Anatomically, the hypothalamus is located just above the brainstem and beneath the thalamus, forming the ventral part of the diencephalon. The nuclei of the hypothalamus integrate information from higher brain regions and visceral and interoceptive information from the medulla to regulate and integrate endocrine, physiological and behavioural functions.

The hypothalamus is closely connected to the hypophysis or pituitary gland where hormones are released into the bloodstream in order to take their effect on target endocrine glands (for example the adrenal cortex) or tissue. The release of hormones is regulated by negative feedback, demonstrating the reciprocal influence of the nervous and endocrine sytems: The hormones released by the various endocrine glands feed back to the hypothalamus and the pituitary, leading to reduced secretory activity. The interaction between the nervous system and the endocrine systems is not limited to the immediate control of the blood concentration of hormones. Hormones also play a major role in the pre- and perinatal development of the nervous system. For example, steroid hormones have sex-specific effects on the organization of the nervous system in the fetus that lead to differential behavioural effects during later development (Phoenix *et al.*, 1959). And it has also been shown that prenatal exposure to stress hormones such as adrenaline or cortisol can have profound effects on the functioning of the hypothalamic–pituitary axis later in life in humans (e.g. Van den Bergh *et al.*, 2005).

The development of psychoneuroendocrinology

Similar to the reciprocal relation between hormones and behaviour, there is a reciprocal influence between mind and hormones – and psychoneuroendocrinology has evolved by investigating both directions. For many years it has been known that dysfunctions of the endocrine glands are associated with psychiatric illness. For example, as early as the nineteenth century patients suffering from a hypofunction of the adrenal cortex were observed to display psycho-pathological functioning, such as mind-wandering or symptoms of depression (for an account, see, for example, Reus, 1987). But in the first half of the twentieth century it also became apparent that psychological states and psychiatric disorders were associated with altered endocrine functioning. Two important findings sparked a vast number of investigations. Walter B Cannon postulated in 1915 that an organism uses its regulatory mechanisms to maintain physiological stability or homeostasis in the presence of environmental stimuli challenging that stability (for a review on Cannon see Fleming, 1984). Cannon found that these stimuli, which he called 'stresses and strains', can constitute physical, physiological as well as psychological stimuli. These stimuli force an immediate but non-specific endocrine response, the release of adrenaline (also called epinephrine). This physiologic response was termed the 'fight or flight response', because it activates and prepares the organism to produce either behaviour: adrenaline increases the heart rate, blood pressure, respiration and blood flow to skeletal muscles.

The concept of stress on the one hand and a non-specific physiological response to stress was followed but also expanded by Hans Selye (1936, 1956). He found that when rats were exposed to 'nocuous agents' or stressors such as injections of tissue extracts or saline solutions, exposure to extreme temperature, hunger or haemorrhage, a non-specific endocrine event occurred: the release of glucocorticoids from the adrenal cortex. Based on these findings he developed his theory of a 'general adaptation syndrome'. It postulates that organisms cope with stressors through three stages: the *alarm reaction*, in which the stressor and the challenge to homeostasis is detected, the *resistance stage*, during which actual coping occurs, mediated especially by the secretion of glucocorticoids, and an *exhaustion stage*, during which the physiological response is terminated due to an exhaustion of the system, leading to illness or even death.

The work conducted by Cannon and, especially, Selye elicited a vast number of studies that were summarized in 1968 by John Mason in a paper that might be considered the initiation of psychoneuroendocrinology (see Ursin, 1998). Mason reviewed over 200 reports of animal studies, experimental studies of humans exposed to stress in the laboratory or field and studies with psychiatric patients which investigated the impact of psychological stimuli on the activity of the hypothalamus–pituitary–adrenal axis. This review resulted in the postulation of eight principles of psychoneuroendocrinology that still hold today (Ursin, 1998), the first of which reads: 'Psychological influences are among the most potent natural stimuli known to affect pituitary–adrenal cortical activity' (Mason, 1968, p. 596). This observation also meant that the effect of physical or physiological stimuli on the endocrine system is mediated by psychological processes that evaluate or 'appraise' the stimuli.

Psychoneuroendocrinology and stress

The concept of stress is still at the core of psychoneuroendocrinology today. Stress, coping and physiological and psychological damage resulting from stress have been researched profoundly in recent years. In terms of stress, several definitions have been developed. These focus either on stress as the initiating situation, the processes of appraisal, the physiological reaction or even the coping mechanism. A current trend in the research into psychoneuroendocrinology and stress is the integration of both cognitive and physiological aspects into one theoretical model. In this vein, stress is defined as being 'operationalized by stimuli ("stressors"), subjective reports of an experience (humans only), a general non-specific increase in arousal (activation), and the feedback to the brain from this response' (Ursin and Eriksen, 2004, p. 570).

Stressor, stress experience, stress response and feedback are the four main aspects of the Cognitive Activation Theory of Stress (CATS; Ursin and Eriksen, 2004). This theory is based on the assumption that expectancy and predictability of an upcoming stressor or its outcome work as moderators (filter in the brain) between the stressor and the stress response, which is defined as a general activation of the physiological system. Expectancy is defined as the learnt information about the relation between stimuli and responses (stimulus expectancy) or outcomes and responses (outcome expectancy; Ursin and Eriksen, 2004). These expectancies of stimuli and outcome can be either positive (coping), neutral (helplessness) or negative (hopelessness). Ursin (1998) reports in his review that situations in which an individual has the felt ability to cope with the given situation (internal locus of control, sensu Rotter, 1975) lead to a reduced activation of the physiological system (stress response). In CATS, this is defined as a positive outcome expectancy. On the other hand, a lack of control (neutral or negative outcome expectancy) produces a distinct physiological activation (stress response) because the individual is alarmed by the discrepancy between what is expected from a given stimulus and outcome and what actually happens.

The second moderator to the stress response is predictability. Just as a highly probable or a highly improbable stimulus produces a lower activation level, uncertainty produces high arousal (Ursin and Eriksen, 2004). However, within all predictability also lies the affective note – a highly predictable but unattractive stimulus (e.g. a predictable event which is associated with anxiety, as in competitive anxiety for example) potentially produces a high stress response as well.

With regard to all stress responses in CATS, there is a distinction between train and strain. Depending on the expectancy and predictability of an individual, stress responses either 'train' the organism or they are potentially damaging to the organism. This strain may accumulate over a longer period. In this sense, allostasis and allostatic load are currently being discussed, advancing both Cannon's idea of homeostasis and Selye's stage of exhaustion within the general adaptation syndrome.

Usually, physiological reactions adapt to stress. For example, first-time parachutists show a distinct hormonal stress reaction in anticipation of their first jump but this hormonal response levels off after several jumps (Deinzer *et al.*, 1997). However, if chronic stressors impact on the individual, a state of dyshomeostasis develops, which is known as allostasis. Allostasis means 'maintaining stability (homeostasis) through change' (McEwen, 2003, p. 200) and is the outcome from physiological and behavioural responses (stress responses) initiated by the brain which perceived a stimulus as stressful (McEwen, 2003, p. 32). Allostasis may accumulate (allostatic load) and may lead to damage to organs (see McEwen, 2004). In this vein, Selye's (1956) idea of a 'stage of exhaustion' as part of the general adaptation syndrome has also come to be questioned. Despite the phenomenal validity of a low level of stress hormones after prolonged or repeated stress, several observations, such as hypertrophy of the adrenals in stressed animals, contradict an exhaustion (e.g. Bassett and Cairncross, 1975). More importantly, a low level of stress hormones may be the effect of different mechanisms at different levels of the endocrine system. For example, it has been postulated that hypocortisolism associated with stress-related disorders may be the result of reduced biosynthesis or release, a downregulation of the receptors or an enhanced negative feedback sensitivity (cf. Fries *et al.*, 2005).

Psychoneuroendocrinology – a conceptual model

There are generally two routes into studying psychoneuroendocrinology, one examining the effects *of* the endocrine system on behaviour and psychological variables, the other examining the effects *on* the endocrine system by behaviour and psychological variables. Within each route, a quasi-experimental or correlational and an experimental approach can be distinguished. When examining the effects of hormones, correlational studies compare, for example, the behaviour of patients suffering from endocrine dysfunctions with healthy controls, or they compare people during different stages within their hormonal cycles. Experimentally, the effect of hormones is investigated through the application of substances – either hormones or substances that stimulate or block their activity. When examining the effects on the endocrine system by psychological variables or behaviour, a correlational approach compares levels of hormones between groups with different personality traits or compares groups that are exposed to chronic psychosocial conditions, such as the workplace. These psychosocial conditions may also be manipulated experimentally to elicit particular psychological states (e.g. anxiety or stress), or behaviour may be manipulated, for example, by requiring participants to exercise vigorously.

Independent of the approach, when studying the reciprocal influence of hormones and behaviour or psychological variables it needs to be remembered that this influence is neither deterministic nor direct. Hormones only increase the likelihood of a certain behaviour and increase action tendencies. This is because behaviour is constrained by various external factors. Mating behaviour, for example, can only be shown by a rooster in the presence of a hen, but mating behaviour is also less likely when the rooster's primary need is getting food. Thus, the relation between hormones and behaviour is also mediated by internal factors. The most important among those mediators is the CNS. External and internal stimuli are processed and evaluated, leading to further physiologic responses (e.g. the secretion of hormones), psychological responses (e.g. feelings) or behavioural responses (e.g. movement). When studying psychoneuroendocrinology it is important to bear in mind these reciprocal, non-deterministic and indirect influences, and they can be described in a conceptual model of psychoneuroendocrinology (Figure 1.1) that in its original form described the analysis of behavioural neuroendocrinology (Nelson, 2005, p. 17).

The conceptual model shows that the endocrine system is under the control of the CNS. The effects on the secretion of hormones are mediated by the activity of the CNS, especially the hypothalamus. Furthermore, the model demonstrates that hormones do not have a direct influence on behaviour but that they may affect the input level or sensory system (i.e. how stimuli in the environment are

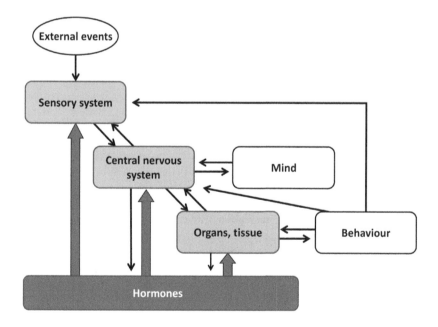

Figure 1.1 A conceptual model of psychoneuroendocrinology highlighting the multiple interactions between the brain as the main moderator, behaviour and hormones.

perceived), they may affect the process level or CNS (i.e. how stimuli are processed) and they may affect output level or the effectors, including organs. Finally, the model also shows that the effect of behaviour on the endocrine system is mediated by the behavioural effects on the sensory system, the CNS and the effectors. Consequently, when one wants to investigate the effects of hormones on behaviour or psychological variables, one needs to address at what level of the model the effects are expected to take place. And when the effect of psychological variables or behaviour on hormones is investigated, it should be considered whether this effect is immediately on the CNS or whether it might be in turn mediated by the sensory system or the effectors.

Psychoneuroendocrinology of sport and exercise

Within sport psychology, the dominant route to studying psychoneuroendocrinology is studying the effects *on* the endocrine system. Many of the studies are correlational in nature or use a design that does not allow a strict determination of causes and effects. For example, aggressive behaviour in sport has often been found to be correlated with higher levels of testosterone (e.g. Salvador *et al.*, 1999) and some studies show that winners of a sports competition have higher levels of testosterone than losers (e.g. Mazur and Lamb, 1980, but see Salvador and Costa, 2009, for a critical review). Another line of research studying the effects of sport behaviour on the endocrine system, although for the most part similarly correlational in nature, has investigated the effects of physical fitness on the endocrine stress response. The so-called 'cross-stressor adaptation hypothesis' postulates that physical fitness should lead to a reduced neuroendocrine stress response (e.g. Gerber, 2008). Consequently, studies have found that people who are more physically active or fit also show a reduced stress response to, for example, cognitive stressors (e.g. Boutcher *et al.*, 1995).

However, not only are the overall results less clear (see e.g. Sothman, 2006; Gerber, 2008; see also Chapter 8), but to understand the causal mechanism behind such a potential adaptive effect, longitudinal and experimental studies are needed with a controlled manipulation of the sports intervention. In general, endocrinological studies show an intensity-dependent activity of the endocrine system in response to an acute bout of physical exercise (e.g. Kjaer, 1992; Dishman and Jackson, 2000). Experimental studies indicate that such an acute bout of exercise also alleviates the physiological response to a psychosocial stressor (see review in Boutcher and Hamer, 2006) but the psychoneuroendocrine mechanism has not received attention. Further studies investigating the effects of sport on the endocrine system have used a time-to-event paradigm by assessing the endocrine stress response in anticipation of sport competition (see for reviews Ehrlenspiel *et al.*, 2008; see also Chapter 7).

There is clearly less research in sport psychology concerned with the effects *of* the endocrine system, at least experimental studies, because the administration of hormones is of ethical concern and in the field of competitive sports, hormones are banned substances. In this vein, however, there have been few (quasi-experimental and correlational) studies that have investigated the psychological side-effects of the abuse of primarily androgenic hormones to enhance sport performance (e.g. Pagonis *et al.*, 2006; for overview, see Bahrke, 2000). Also the research on overtraining and overreaching in sport is concerned with the interaction of exercise, psychological states and the endocrine system, with some research aimed at identifying valid endocrine predictors of the phenomenon (e.g. Coutts *et al.*, 2007; see also Chapter 10).

The psychoneuroendocrinological approach to sport psychology is obviously confronted with a number of difficulties. It appears that sport may not be well suited for the investigation of basic mechanisms in the interaction of brain, hormones and behaviour or mind. Invasive methods that either manipulate the endocrine system via substances or that assess hormones in the blood or even in the CNS are difficult to apply. This is both because of ethical considerations and because invasive methods should themselves be considered a manipulation (or intervention) that induce stress. It is also because of the practical difficulties in applying these techniques in the field setting in which many sport psychology questions arise and are investigated. This field setting also impairs the control of important constraints and confounding factors. Lastly, for the identification of basic mechanisms, the observation of the interaction between brain and hormones should include the analysis of this interaction at the level of the brain. Thus, although one might find it appealing that certain ideas about basic psychoneuroendocrine mechanisms are also shown to hold in sport – for example the relation between aggression and testosterone – sport may still not be the optimal test bed for the study of these basic psychoneuroendocrine mechanisms.

In addition, it might be asked whether it is the place of sport psychology or sport psychologists to develop or to test these mechanisms, even if they could be tested in sport. To define the objective of a psychoneuroendocrinology of sport and exercise, we need to turn to the beginning of this chapter, in which we laid out what sport psychology is concerned with in general. Here we stated that the study of human behaviour and experience in sport is interested in the analysis of the effects of the mind on sport and in the analysis of the effects of sport on the mind. The objective of a psychoneuroendocrinology of sport and exercise now arises from the need to find physiological mechanisms that can explain these effects. Psychoneuroendocrinology is one among other areas of (psycho-)biology that could and should provide us with insights into these mechanisms. In following this objective, psychoneuroendocrinology would also play an important role in the much needed integration of the various orientations within sport psychology with a biological orientation (as Acevedo and Ekkekakis, 2006b, demanded). Psychoneuroendocrinology of sport should avoid 'scientism' – simply demonstrating the reciprocal effects between the mind and the endocrine system, most often in some correlative design. Rather it should assist in the full understanding of (psychological) phenomena in sport by providing insights into their physiological mechanism, thereby also avoiding a 'dualism' between mind and body.

Recently, some studies that have generally followed this integrative path and that go beyond simply testing the effects of or on the endocrine system in sport have been published. They can be perceived as attempts to find a psychoneuroendocrine mechanism behind a phenomenon, an observation or a theory from the social–psychological or the cognitive behavioural orientation of sport psychology.

Investigating a well-known social–psychological phenomenon, the 'home advantage' in competitive sport (e.g. Jamieson, 2010, Strauß and Bierschwale, 2008), Carré and co-workers (2006) assessed hormones before home and away games in hockey. They found that players exhibited both increased levels of testosterone and cortisol before home games, but also increased anxiety before away games. Thus they link the home advantage to a reaction of the endocrine system that provides the organism with more activation (testosterone) and energy (cortisol). Other studies have investigated the effects of competition on performance from a psychoneuroendocrine perspective. In a laboratory study a simulated competition led to enhanced performance in an all-out treadmill exercise compared to a non-competition baseline (Viru *et al.*, 2010). In addition, while the exercise generally led to increases in concentrations of testosterone and growth hormone, only after the competition was the concentration of cortisol elevated.

A further study found somewhat contradictory results. Even in anticipation of the competition higher concentrations of cortisol were found in tennis players who lost a match early in a tournament (Filaire *et al.*, 2009). Thus although the findings appear inconclusive at this stage, all of these studies attempt to provide a psychoneuroendocrine mechanism for prominent phenomena of a social–psychology orientation in sport psychology.

A similar observation can be made for the cognitive behavioural orientation: 'The empirical evidence for a neuroendocrinological rationale for an acute exercise–cognitive function interaction is weak' (McMorris, 2009, p. 63) and, it may be added, inconclusive. For example, in a study with adolescents, a positive effect of a short physical exercise on cognitive function was observed only when baseline performance was poor. On the other hand, increase of testosterone as an effect of more intense exercising was also associated with poorer performance (Budde *et al.*, 2010). Despite this empirical weakness, complex models of the neuroendocrinological mechanism showing the effect of exercise on cognitive functioning have recently been developed that allow empirical scrutiny (McMorris, 2009).

Also within the cognitive behavioural orientation it is assumed that physical exercise has positive effects on mood and affective disorders (e.g. Wipfli *et al.*, 2008). Although there are a number of hypotheses on the mechanism of this effect, few studies have investigated the role of hormones. For example, a hormone produced in the heart, atrial natriuretic peptide, has been found to have anxiolytic effects and is also elevated after physical exercise, suggesting a mediating role (Ströhle *et al.*, 2006).

With regard to these examples from the social and the cognitive behavioural orientation, we find that although the results are far from conclusive and to some degree also lack a clear reference to a psychological theory, they still indicate what a psychoneuroendocrinology of sport and exercise should be concerned with: identifying the mediating processes involved in the effects of mind on sport and of sport on the mind.

This volume is aimed at facilitating research in psychoneuroendocrinology and helping to fill the void of research integrating the more psychological orientations in sport psychology with a psycho-biological orientation. In following the belief that this integration of 'mind and body' in sport must happen in sport psychology by sport psychologists we intend to provide a foundation for psychoneuroendocrinology of sport and exercise. To this end, an introductory chapter (Chapter 2) not only presents the idea of a psychoneuroendocrinology of sport and exercise, but also gives an introduction to the basic concepts and terms. This introduction will allow readers to understand the second section (Part II), in which the most important markers for a psychoneuroendocrinology of sport and exercise are introduced. Keeping in mind that methods should be applicable in sport psychology, we have focused on markers that can be assessed by non-invasive methods. In Part III we present current research in the field.

References

Acevedo, E. O. and Ekkekakis, P. (eds) (2006a). *Psychobiology of Physical Activity*. Champaign, IL: Human Kinetics.

Acevedo, E. O. and Ekkekakis, P. (2006b). Psychobiology of physical activity: integration at last. In E. O. Acevedo and P. Ekkekakis (eds), *Psychobiology of Physical Activity* (pp. 1–14). Champaign, IL: Human Kinetics.

Anshel, M. (2003). *Sport Psychology: from Theory To Practice*, 4th edn. San Francisco: Benjamin–Cummings.

Bahrke, M. S. (2000). Psychological effects of endogenous testosterone and anabolic-androgenic steroids. In C. E. Yesalis (ed.), *Anabolic Steroids in Sport and Exercise*, 2nd edn (pp. 247–278). Champaign, IL: Human Kinetics.

Bar-Eli, M. and Blumenstein, B. (2004). Performance enhancement in swimming: the effect of mental training with biofeedback. *Journal of Science and Medicine in Sport*, 7, 454–464.

Bassett, J. R. and Cairncross, K. D. (1975). Morphological changes induced in rats following prolonged exposure to stress. *Pharmacology, Biochemistry and Behavior*, 3, 411–420.

Becker, J. B. and Breedlove, S. M. (2002). Introduction to behavioral endocrinology. In J. B. Becker, S. M. Breedlove, D. Crews and M. M. McCarthy (eds), *Behavioral Endocrinology*, 2nd edn (pp. 3–38). Cambridge, MA: MIT Press.

Beilock, S. L. and Carr, T. H. (2001). On the fragility of skilled performance: what governs choking under pressure? *Journal of Experimental Psychology: General*, 130, 701–725.

Boutcher S. H. and Hamer M. (2006). Psychobiological reactivity, physical activity, and cardiovascular health. In E. O. Acevedo and P. Ekkekakis (eds), *Psychobiology of Physical Activity* (pp. 161–176). Champaign, IL: Human Kinetics.

Boutcher, S. H., Nugent, F. W. and Weltman, A. L. (1995). Heart rate response to psychological stressors of individuals possessing resting bradycardia. *Behavioral Medicine*, 21, 40–46.

Budde, H., Voelcker-Rehage, C., Pietrassyk-Kendziorra, S., Machado, S., Ribeiro, P. and Arafat, A. M. (2010). Steroid hormones in the saliva of adolescents after different exercise intensities and their influence on working memory in a school setting. *Psychoneuroendocrinology*. 35, 382–391.

Burke, S. M., Carron, A. V. and Shapcott, K. M. (2008). Cohesion in exercise groups: an overview. *International Review of Sport and Exercise Psychology*, 1, 107–123.

Cannon, W. B. (1929). *Bodily Changes in Pain, Hunger, Fear and Rage*. New York: Appleton.

Carré, J. M., Muir, C., Belanger, J. and Putnam, SK. (2006). Pre-competition hormonal and psychological levels of elite hockey players: relationship to the home advantage. *Physiology and Behavior*, 30, 392–398.

Carron, A. V., Colman, M. M., Wheeler, J. and Stevens, D. (2002). Cohesion and performance in sport: a meta analysis. *Journal of Sport and Exercise Psychology*, 24, 168–188.

Chiviakowsky, S., Wulf, G. and Wally, R. (2010). An external focus of attention enhances balance learning in older adults. *Gait and Posture*, 32, 572–575.

Council of Europe (2001). Committee of Ministers, Recommendation No. R (92) 13 REV of the Committee of Ministers to Member States on the revised European Sports Charter. http://wcd.coe.int/ViewDoc.jsp?Ref=Rec(92)13 (retrieved 23 February 2011).

Coutts, A.J., Reaburn, P., Piva, T. and Rowsell, G. (2007). Monitoring for overreaching in rugby league players. *European Journal of Applied Physiology*, 99, 313–324.

Crabbe, J. B. and Dishman, R. K. (2004). Brain electrocortical activity during and after exercise: a quantitative synthesis. *Psychophysiology*, 41, 563–574.

Craft, L. L., Magyar, T. M., Becker, B. J. and Feltz, D. L. (2003). The relationship between the competitive state anxiety inventory-2 and sport performance: a meta-analysis. *Journal of Sport and Exercise Psychology*, 25, 44–65.

Deinzer, R., Kirschbaum, C., Gresele, C. and Hellhammer, D. H. (1997). Adrenocortical responses to repeated parachute jumping and subsequent h-CRH challenge in inexperienced healthy subjects. *Physiology and Behavior*, 61, 507–511.

Dishman, R. K. (1994). Biological psychology, exercise and stress. *Quest*, 46, 39–47.

Dishman R. K. and Jackson, E. M. (2000). Exercise, fitness, and stress. *International Journal of Sport Psychology*, 31, 175–203.

Dosseville, F., Laborde, S. and Raab, M. (2011). Contextual and personal motor experience. Effects in judo referees' decisions. *The Sport Psychologist*, 25, 67–81.

Ehrlenspiel, F., Beckmann, J.and Strahler, K. (2008). Competitive anxiety – review and perspectives with a neuroendocrine slant. In A. Blachnio and A. Przepiórka (eds), *Blizej emocji II [Closer to emotions]* (pp. 166-183). Lublin: Wydawtniktwo KUL.

Ehrlenspiel, F., Wei, K. and Sternad, D. (2010). Open-loop, closed-loop, and compensatory control: performance under pressure in a rhythmic task. *Experimental Brain Research*, 201, 729–741.,

Erickson, K. I. and Kramer, A. F. (2009). Aerobic exercise effects on cognitive and neural plasticity in older adults. *British Journal of Sports Medicine*, 43, 22–24.

Filaire, E., Maso, F., Sagnol, M., Ferrand, C. and Lac, G. (2001). Anxiety, hormonal responses, and coping during a judo competition. *Aggressive Behavior*, 27, 55–63.

Filaire, E., Alix, D., Ferrand, C. and Verger, M. (2009). Psychophysiological stress in tennis players during the first single match of a tournament. *Psychoneuroendocrinology*, 34, 150–157.

Fleming, D. (1984). Walter B. Cannon and homeostasis. *Social Research*, 51, 609–640.

Fries, E., Hesse, J., Hellhammer, J. and Hellhammer, D. (2005). A new view on hypocortisolism. *Psychoneuroendocrinology*, 30, 1010–1016.

Gerber, M. (2008). Sportliche aktivität und stressreaktivität: ein review. [Exercise and stress reactivity: a review]. *Deutsche Zeitschrift für Sportmedizin*, 59, 168–174.

Gill, D. L. (2000). *Psychological Dynamics of Sport and Exercise*, 2nd edn. Champaign, IL: Human Kinetics.

Hanin, Y. L. (2000). Individual zones of optimal functioning. In Y. L. Hanin (ed.), *Emotions in Sport* (pp. 65–89). Champaign, IL: Human Kinetics.

Hatfield, B. D. and Landers, D. M. (1983). Psychophysiology – A new direction for sport psychology. *Journal of Sport Psychology*, 5, 243–259.

Jamieson, J. P. (2010). The home field advantage in athletics: a meta-analysis. *Journal of Applied Social Psychology*, 40, 1819–1848.

Kjaer, M. (1992). Regulation of hormonal and metabolic responses during exercise in humans. *Exercise and Sport Science Review*, 20, 161–184.

Mason, J. (1968). A review of psychoendocrine research on the pituitary-adrenal cortical system. *Psychosomatic Medicine*, 30, 576–607.

Mazur, A. and Lamb, T.A., (1980). Testosterone, status and mood in human males. *Hormones and Behavior*, 14, 236–246.

McCubbin, J.A. (2000). Psychoneuroendocrinology. In A. E. Kazdin (ed.), *Encyclopedia of Psychology* (pp. 420–423). New York: Oxford University Press.

McEwen, B. S. (2003). Mood disorders and allostatic load. *Biological Psychiatry*, 54, 200–207.

McEwen, B. S. (2004). Protection and damage from acute and chronic stress: allostasis and allostatic overload and relevance to the pathophysiology of psychiatric disorders. *Annals of the New York Academy of Sciences*, 1032, 1–7.

McMorris, T. (2009). Exercise and cognitive function: a neuroendocrinological explanation. In T. McMorris, P. Tomporowski and M. Audiffren (eds), *Exercise and Cognitive Function* (pp. 41–68). Chichester: Wiley-Blackwell.

Morris, T., Alfermann, D., Lintunen, T. and Hall, H. (2003). Training and selection of sport psychologists: an international review. *International Journal of Sport and Exercise Psychology*, 1, 139–154.

Nelson, R. J. (2005). *An Introduction to Behavioral Endocrinology*, 3rd edn. Sunderland, MA: Sinauer.

Pagonis, T. A., Angelopoulos, N. V., Koukoulis, G. N. and Hadjichristodoulou, C. S. (2006). Psychiatric side effects induced by supraphysiological doses of combinations of anabolic steroids correlate to the severity of abuse. *European Psychiatry*, 21, 551–562.

Phoenix, C., Goy, R. W., Gerall, A. A. and Young, W. C. (1959). Organizing action of prenatally administered testosterone proprionate on the tissues mediating behaviour in the female guinea pig. *Endocrinology*, 65, 369–382.

Reus, V. I. (1987). Disorders of the adrenal cortex and gonads. In C. B. Nemeroff and P. T. Loosen (eds), *Handbook of Clinical Psychoneuroendocrinology* (pp. 71–84). New York: Guilford Press.

Rotter, J. B. (1975). Some problems and misconceptions related to the construct of internal versus external control of reinforcement. *Journal of Consulting and Clinical Psychology*, 43, 56–67.

Salvador, A. and Costa, R. (2009). Coping with competition: neuroendocrine responses and cognitive variables. *Neurosciences and Biobehavioral Reviews*, 33, 160–170.

Salvador, A., Suay, F., Martinez-Sanchis, S., Simon, V. M., Brain, P. F. (1999). Correlating testosterone and fighting in male participants in judo contests. *Physiological Behavior*, 68, 205–209.

Selye, H. (1936). A syndrome produced by diverse nocuous agents. *Nature*, 138, 32–35.

Selye, H. (1956). *The Stress of Life*. New York: McGraw-Hill.

Sothman, M. S. (2006). The cross-stressor adaptation hypothesis and exercise training. In E. Acevedo and P. Ekkekakis (eds), *Psychobiology of Physical Activity* (pp. 145–160). Champaign, IL: Human Kinetics.

Strauß, B. and Bierschwale, J. (2008). Zuschauer und der heimvorteil in der handball-bundesliga [Spectators and the home advantage in the german national handball league]. *Zeitschrift für Sportpsychologie*, 15, 96–101.

Ströhle, A., Feller, C., Strasburger, C. J., Heinz, A. and Dimeo, F. (2006). Anxiety modulation by the heart? Aerobic exercise and atrial natriuretic peptide. *Psychoneuroendocrinology*, 31, 1127–1130.

Szymanski, B., Beckmann, J., Elbe, A.-M. and Müller, D. (2004). Wie entwickelt sich die volition bei talenten an einer eliteschule des sports? [How does volition develop in students at school for talented young athletes?]. *Zeitschrift für Sportpsychologie*, 11, 103–111.

Triplett, N. (1898). The dynamogenic factors in pacemaking and competition. *American Journal of Psychology*, 9, 507–533.

Ursin, H. (1998). The psychology in psychoneuroendocrinology. *Psychoneuroendocrinology*, 23, 555–570.

Ursin, H. and Eriksen, H. R. (2004). The cognitive activation theory of stress. *Psychoneuroendocrinology*, 29, 567–592.

Van den Bergh, B. R. H., Mulder, E. J. H., Mennes, M. and Glover, V. (2005). Antenatal maternal anxiety and stress and the neurobehavioural development of the fetus and child: links and possible mechanisms. A review. *Neuroscience and Biobehavioral Reviews*, 29, 237–258.

Viru, M., Hackney, A. C., Karelson, K., Janson, T., Kuus, M. and Viru, A. (2010). Competition effects on physiological responses to exercise: performance, cardiorespiratory and hormonal factors. *Acta Physiologica Hungarica*, 97, 22–30.

Weinberg, R. and Gould, D. (2003). *Foundations of Sport and Exercise Psychology*, 3rd edn. Champaign, IL: Human Kinetics.

Wipfli, B. M., Rethorst, C. D. and Landers, D. (2008). The anxiolytic effects of exercise: a meta-analysis of randomized trials and dose–response analysis. *Journal of Sport and Exercise Psychology*, 30, 392–410.

Woodman, T. and Hardy, L. (2003). The relative impact of cognitive anxiety and self-confidence upon sport performance: a meta-analysis. *Journal of Sports Sciences*, 21, 443–457.

Yerkes, R. M. and Dodson, J. D. (1908). The relation of strength of stimulus to rapidity of habit-formation. *Journal of Comparative Neurology and Psychology*, 18, 459–482.

2 Foundations in psychoneuroendocrinology

Jana Strahler and Elisabeth Klumbies

This chapter provides an introduction to psychoneuroendocrinology. Assuming a general understanding of basic concepts in neurobiology, the basic concepts of neuroendocrinology are provided, such as hormonal communication and the basics of signal transduction. The role of the hypothalamus and the hypothalamic–pituitary relations in the regulation of hormones are described, and an overview on the endocrine glands and the types of hormones they secrete is provided. To lay the ground for the following chapters, emphasis is given to hormones of the anterior pituitary and of the adrenal glands as well as to androgens. A short overview of the techniques used in the study of psychoneuroendocrinology is also provided, with a focus on stimulation and suppression.

Psychoneuroendocrinology: definition

Reports from athletes' everyday life commonly highlight the close connection between endocrine systems and psychological processes. It is common knowledge that physical exercise is able to produce positive emotions, such as feelings of euphoria mediated via increases of endogenous β-endorphin ('runner's high'), and that in anticipation of a competition, psychological processes such as nervousness or fear of failure are able to induce a physiological hyperactivity (e.g. increased heart rate, faster breathing, increased sweating and changes in hormonal levels), which might consequently lead to poorer sport performance.

These and other phenomena are the research focus of psychoneuroendocrinology. This branch of research originated in the 1950s following reports of endocrine disorders being associated with clinically relevant psychological disorders such as psychotic disorders. The overall aim of psychoneuroendocrinology research is the identification of biological markers of mental health problems based on the assumption of a strong relation between stressful experiences and disorders mediated via a stress-induced dysregulation of the endocrine system. Psychoneuroendocrinology investigates interrelations between the mind (i.e. behaviour) and experience, as well as the central nervous system (CNS) and endocrine system functioning.

(1) Psychoneuroendocrinology assesses the impact of hormones on the mind:

- via the experimental manipulation of hormones (application, stimulation, blocking) such as the investigation of exercise-related changes of depressive symptoms or
- on a correlative basis, by comparing patients suffering from hormonal dysfunctions and healthy controls or subjects during different phases of hormonal regulation (e.g. during the menstrual cycle).

(2) Psychoneuroendocrinology assesses the impact of the mind on hormone levels:

- via the effects of manipulating psychological states (e.g. inducing psychological stress, performance tasks, positive emotions, social interaction, but also sleeping, eating and sexual behaviour) on hormonal alterations or
- by comparing subjects with different personality characteristics or under different psychosocial conditions, such as investigating stress hormones during training versus competition (keywords 'choking under pressure').

Biological basics

The endocrine system

The endocrine system comprises all hormone-producing organs and cells. It signals information via hormones (from the Greek *hormon*, to excite) as extracellular messengers that regulate body functions and thus control behaviour. Hormones are secreted by the endocrine glands into the bloodstream (diffusion) and transported to their effector organs. The main hormonal functions are growth and development (e.g. thyroid hormones, growth hormone), reproduction (e.g. oestrogen, testosterone) and homeostasis (e.g. thyroid hormones, cortisol). Hormones are classified into protein or peptide hormones (e.g. thyroid-stimulating hormone (TSH) and insulin), monoamines (e.g. adrenaline) and steroid hormones (e.g. cortisol) (Table 2.1).

Table 2.1 Classification of hormones

Hormone class	Structure	Examples
Peptide or protein hormones	Largest class of hormones; peptide hormones consist of amino acid sequences of varying length; proteins composed of long chains of amino acids (>100) are referred to as protein hormones	Thyroid-releasing hormone and vasopressin, insulin and growth hormone
Monoamines	Smallest class of hormones; amino hormones consist of only one amino acid modified by specific enzymes	(Nor)adrenaline and thyroxin
Steroid hormones	Cholesterol-derived hormones; fat-soluble and thus able to pass through the cell membrane	Testosterone, oestrogens, and glucocorticoids

Biological rhythms

The main regulators of hormonal secretion are biological rhythms, sleep and responses to exogenous events. There is no stable basal value but rather a secretory dynamic of hormone production. These rhythms permeate all levels of biological activity, from gene expression and hormone secretion to behaviour such as cognitive ability. There are various kinds of endogenous rhythms, including circadian rhythms, seasonal rhythms, lunar rhythms and lifetime rhythms, as described below.

Many aspects of human life undergo distinct alterations throughout the 24-hour cycle, so-called *circadian rhythms*. These rhythms are thought to be regulated by environmental factors and generated by the suprachiasmatic nucleus which is located in the hypothalamus. This nucleus receives photic input from retinal cells and projects to multiple organs of the body, including parts of the endocrine system. Endocrine parameters that are characterized by a pronounced circadian rhythmicity are the glucocorticoid cortisol and the sleep-dependent secretion of growth hormone. Another hormone that is synchronized to the 24-hour cycle by cues from the light–dark cycle is melatonin. Under normal circumstances, melatonin is produced during the night and exposure to light inhibits melatonin.

Importantly, melatonin secretion is not only adjusted to the light–dark cycle itself, but is also known to be positively related to the length of the night. Thus, the secretion pattern of melatonin also serves as a cue for *seasonal rhythms*.

Other hormones are released in a *pulsatile manner*, such as luteinizing hormone (LH) and TSH. Under normal circumstances, these hormones are released in pulses of 90–120 minutes. The monthly variation of hormones such as oestrogen and progesterone during the menstrual cycle is called *lunar rhythm*. *Lifetime rhythms* are exemplified by the release of growth hormone, which has high values during puberty and a sharp decline thereafter, or testosterone, which is known to be at its highest levels during the mid twenties and steadily decreases afterwards.

Hormonal signal transduction

As already noted, cells of the endocrine system are able to communicate by releasing hormones as chemical signals. Typically, several steps comprise this signalling. The process begins with the synthesis and release of the hormone into the bloodstream. Then it is transported to the target cell and a specific receptor detects the hormone. In general, there are two types of hormone receptors that are based on a lock and key principle. The first mode describes signalling via intracellular receptors that lead to the uptake of hormones into the target cell. Second, the binding of hormones on plasma membrane receptors activates an intracellular signal, the second messenger cyclic adenosine monophosphate. Both ways cause a change in cellular metabolism and function. Finally, the signal molecule is removed. This terminates the cellular response within the target cell.

According to their production and target locations, hormonal signalling is classified into three classes: autocrine, paracrine, and endocrine signalling. *Autocrine* signalling describes the effects of hormones that bind to receptors on the releasing cell itself. For instance, during an immune response T cells secrete growth factors to which they themselves respond, start increasing their number and thus help trigger an effective immune response. Signalling in which the target cell is near the signal-releasing cell is called *paracrine* cell signalling (tissue hormones such as growth hormone, serotonin or prostaglandins). The typical mode of cell signalling is *endocrine* signalling. Endocrine hormones are secreted into the bloodstream and affect cells more distantly located. A special case here is the release of neurohormones by neurons that receive neuronal input (keywords: action potential and neurotransmitter) and release hormones directly into the bloodstream. In this case, one speaks of *neuroendocrine* secretion that brings about integration between the CNS and the endocrine system (Figure 2.1). One typical example is the neuroendocrine cells of the hypothalamus which receive neuronal input and secrete releasing hormones.

Endocrine glands of the central nervous system

Main endocrine glands are the hypothalamus and pituitary

The endocrine systems of the body are mainly operated and integrated via the hypothalamus and pituitary gland that receive their input from the CNS. The hypothalamus contains a number of small nuclei (>30) that are responsible for certain autonomic functions to maintain homeostasis; this includes blood pressure, heart rate, temperature, metabolic processes, reproductive functions and water balance. It synthesizes and secretes various so-called hypothalamic-releasing hormones that stimulate or inhibit pituitary activities. The pituitary gland (also called the hypophysis) is located directly below the hypothalamus. This gland, which is

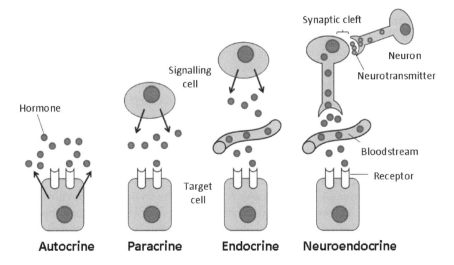

Figure 2.1 Types of intercellular signalling.

about the size of a pea, is responsible for the regulation of the endocrine systems via the secretion of various hormones. It is divided into the anterior pituitary (adenohypophysis), the posterior pituitary (neurohypophysis), and the intermediate lobe. The hypothalamus and pituitary are functionally connected via the eminentia mediana, where axons of hypothalamic neuroendocrine cells end, and via the pituitary stalk that contains many axons and blood vessels and therefore provides the basis for hormonal signal transduction between both endocrine glands.

Together with the neurohypophysis, the organum vasculosum of the lamina terminalis, the subfornical organ and the area postrema, the eminentia mediana is one of the so-called circumventricular organs which are outside the blood–brain barrier. These barrier-deficient structures permit hypothalamic hormones to leave the brain due to the structural vascular specializations that make up the blood–brain barrier (Ganong, 2000).

Release of hormones via the anterior pituitary

Hypothalamic nuclei are easily classified according to their region (anterior, intermediate or posterior) and the area (medial or lateral). Neuroendocrine cells of the medial nuclei regulate the release of hormones within the anterior pituitary. They receive input via two different ways. On the one hand, they receive synaptic input from different brain regions such as the limbic system (hippocampus, amygdala) and the brainstem (locus coeruleus). The limbic system is known for its role in emotion processing. The locus coeruleus is the major source of the central noradrenergic axons which play an important role in the autonomic stress response and vigilance. Thus, human experience and behaviour is able to affect (neuro-)endocrine processes. On the other hand, the hypothalamus is bounded in part by specialized brain regions (e.g. circumventricular organs, as mentioned above) that lack an effective blood–brain barrier. Here, neurons are in close contact with both blood and cerebrospinal fluid, which allows free transfer of even large molecules. Those neurons register blood substances such as hormones, glucose or cytokines and project to the hypothalamus. Thus, hormones in the blood as well as brain-derived neurotransmitters have important regulatory effects on hypothalamic function.

Axons of hypothalamic cells end at the highly vascularized eminentia mediana in the pituitary stalk. There, two different kinds of steering hormones are secreted into the local bloodstream – *releasing hormones* that enhance and *inhibiting hormones* that inhibit the release of hormones from the anterior pituitary. Via the hypophyseal portal system, hypothalamic hormones are distributed to the pituitary where they trigger the release of hormones into the bloodstream.

The anterior pituitary synthesizes and secretes two *effector hormones* (prolactin and growth hormone) and four *trophic hormones* (adrenocorticotrophic hormone (ACTH), TSH, LH and follicle-stimulating hormone (FSH)). Effector hormones directly affect their target cells and organs while trophic hormones act indirectly via the stimulation of other hormones.

In sum, there are up to three intermediate steps from the CNS to the release of effective/operative hormones: the hypothalamus, the pituitary and – in the case of trophic hormones – peripheral endocrine glands. These major peripheral endocrine glands are the adrenal gland, the thyroid gland, ovary or testis and the pancreas. According to the location of the peripheral endocrine glands, specific hormonal axes are differentiated. In the following text these axes are described in detail (see also Figure 2.2).

The hypothalamic–pituitary–adrenal axis

The hypothalamic–pituitary–adrenal (HPA) axis regulates the production and release of corticosteroids from the adrenal cortex. Disruption of homeostasis stimulates the HPA axis and induces the release of corticotrophin-releasing hormone (CRH) from the paraventricular nucleus of the hypothalamus. In conjunction with arginine vasopressin (AVP), CRH stimulates the production of ACTH in the pituitary. This hormone enters the bloodstream and stimulates the release of glucocorticoids (chiefly cortisol in humans) from the adrenal cortex. In turn, glucocorticoids suppress hypothalamic CRH and pituitary ACTH production in a negative feedback loop. In blood, cortisol is bound to binding proteins and

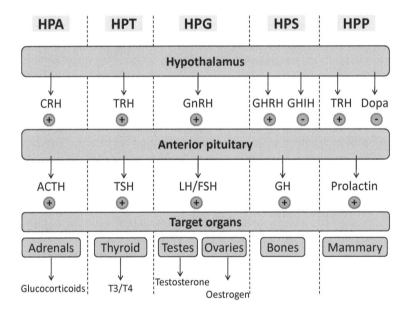

Figure 2.2 Overview of main endocrine axes. HPA, hypothalamic–pituitary–adrenal; HPT, hypothalamic–pituitary–thyroid; HPG, hypothalamic–pituitary–gonadal; HPS, hypothalamic–pituitary–somatrophic; HPP, hypothalamic–pituitary–prolactin; CRH, corticotrophin-releasing hormone; TRH, thyrotrophin-releasing hormone; GnRH, gonadotrophin-releasing hormone; GHRH, growth hormone-releasing hormone; GHIH, growth hormone-inhibiting hormone; Dopa, dopamine; ACTH, adrenocorticotrophic hormone; TSH, thyroid-stimulating hormone; LH, luteinizing hormone; FSH, follicle-stimulating hormone; GH, growth hormone.

therefore only 5–10% of total plasma cortisol is biologically active, the so-called free cortisol.

Free cortisol binds to two different types of intracellular steroid receptors: glucocorticoid and mineralocorticoid receptors. Since those receptors are present in nearly every organ and tissue of the body, cortisol mediates various processes. In short, cortisol stimulates gluconeogenesis and fat breakdown in adipose tissue; it inhibits protein synthesis, glucose uptake in muscle and adipose tissue; and it inhibits immunological and inflammatory responses. Activity of the HPA axis has been studied extensively and it has been shown that its dysfunction is involved in the development and/or progression of various disease states, including the metabolic syndrome, diabetes, hypertension, depression and cognitive impairments (Chrousos and Gold, 1992; Holsboer, 2000; Belanoff *et al.*, 2001; Bjorntorp, 2001).

Since the early 1970s, basal as well as acute stress-induced HPA axis activity has also been examined in athletes. In sum, these studies suggest a reduced HPA axis activation in response to physical (treadmill exercise) and psychological stress in highly trained athletes (e.g. Luger *et al.*, 1987; Rimmele *et al.*, 2007; Rimmele *et al.*, 2009; see also Chapter 8). Furthermore, a mild hypercortisolism was shown under basal conditions and in response to pharmacological stimuli (Luger *et al.*, 1987; Heuser *et al.*, 1991). This might be due to a downregulation of glucocorticoid receptor mRNA expression (Bonifazi *et al.*, 2009). Issues pertaining to exercise and cortisol, as a final effector of the HPA axis, will be reviewed in Chapter 3.

The hypothalamic–pituitary–thyroid axis

The main function of the hypothalamic–pituitary–thyroid (HPT) axis is the regulation of metabolism via the secretion of thyroid hormones. Thyrotrophin-releasing hormone is released from the paraventricular nucleus of the hypothalamus and distributed via the hypophyseal portal system to the pituitary, where it stimulates the synthesis and secretion of TSH. TSH, in turn, is transported via the bloodstream to the thyroid gland and stimulates the production of triiodothyronine (T3) and thyroxin (T4). The thyroid hormones T3 and T4 regulate metabolic functions of proteins, fat, carbohydrates and mineral nutrients, and influence central nervous and reproductive processes. Furthermore, T3 and T4 exert negative feedback control over the hypothalamus as well as the anterior pituitary.

Since thyroid hormones are important regulators of energy metabolism, the function and pathology of the HPT axis has also been investigated in athletes. Decreases in metabolic rate are known to stimulate the HPT axis. Indeed, the effects of exercise on thyroid hormone levels remain controversial. Acute exercise results in an increase of TSH and T4, and a decrease of T3 levels (Ciloglu *et al.*, 2005). This might reflect the relative negative energy balance during acute exercise. On the other hand, chronic exercise is associated with a suppression of peripheral thyroid hormone metabolism (for a review see Mastorakos and Pavlatou, 2005). In contrast, one recent study could not confirm this effect of chronic exercise on thyroid function tests in elite taekwondo fighters (Pilz-Burstein *et al.*, 2010). To date, the significance of exercise-induced changes in thyroid hormone levels has not been fully assessed.

The hypothalamic–pituitary–gonadal axis

The hypothalamic–pituitary–gonadal (HPG) axis controls the function of the gonads and therefore plays a role in development, reproduction and ageing. The nucleus arcuatus and nearby hypothalamic nuclei secrete gonadotrophin-releasing hormone (GnRH) which, in turn, stimulates the synthesis and secretion of FSH and LH from the anterior pituitary. Both hormones are transported to the gonads. In women, the main function of FSH is to control follicle maturation. LH triggers ovulation, and stimulates the formation of the corpus luteum, which produces oestrogen and progesterone. Both hormones therefore control the female's menstrual cycle. In men, LH stimulates the production and release of testosterone in interstitial cells. FSH influences Sertoli cells and, together with testosterone, plays a role in spermatogenesis.

Since the late 1970s, exercise-induced variations in gonadal androgens have often been studied. Acute resistance exercise is known to be associated with a decline in testosterone concentration as well as blunted LH levels (Nindl *et al.*, 2001), while FSH is generally not influenced (Elias and Wilson, 1993). Furthermore, chronic exercise is able to inhibit gonadal functions, possibly due to changes in GnRH pulse frequency and amplitude. There is increasing evidence for so-called 'exercise-related female reproductive dysfunction', including amenorrhoea, infertility, eating disorders, osteoporosis and coronary heart disease (Mastorakos *et al.*, 2005). In men, the 'exercise-hypogonadal male condition' has been the subject of many investigations showing endurance training to be detrimental to reproductive hormone profiles (Hackney, 2008). Chapters 4 and 8 provide an overview of the association between testosterone levels and exercise.

The hypothalamic–pituitary–somatotrophic system

The hypothalamic–pituitary–somatotrophic (HPS) system is responsible for the growth of cells and tissues. The nucleus arcuatus and the nucleus ventromedialis of the hypothalamus secrete growth hormone-releasing hormone (GHRH) which is transported via the hypophyseal portal system into the anterior pituitary. This, in turn, stimulates the secretion of growth hormone. Hypothalamic growth hormone-inhibiting hormone (GHIH, somatostatin) acts antagonistically on GHRH and inhibits the release of growth hormone. The generally anabolic effects of growth hormone include the stimulation of growth, cell reproduction and regeneration (e.g. insulin-like growth factor 1 release from the liver). Growth hormone is released in a pulsatile manner and its secretion rate peaks around sleep onset. It is therefore widely sleep-dependent and is found to be suppressed during sleep deprivation.

The anabolic effects of growth hormone have been thoroughly studied. It is known that exercise stimulates the secretion of serum growth hormone within about 15 minutes after stimulus onset and regular exercise is known to raise basal growth hormone secretion (Widdowson *et al.*, 2009). This might contribute to the physiological alterations seen, such as increased muscle strength and improved body composition. This observation, among others, led to the abuse of growth hormone to increase muscle mass and strength in athletes. However, scientific studies have not confirmed any additional effect of growth hormone treatment on strength in highly trained subjects (Frisch, 1999; Rogol, 2010).

The hypothalamic–pituitary–prolactin axis

The hypothalamic–pituitary–prolactin (HPP) axis has its main effect in reproduction, such as regulating breast development and lactation. Prolactin-releasing factors stimulate the acute release of prolactin from the anterior pituitary. Some of these factors are prolactin-releasing-hormone or prolactoliberin, hypothalamic thyrotrophin-releasing hormone and oxytocin, which are activated by serotonin. Prolactin secretion is also under hypothalamic inhibitory control, mediated via dopamine secreted from tuberohypophyseal dopaminergic neurons. Prolactin is released continuously throughout the day with peaks during night and in the middle of the menstrual cycle. It also increases in response to stress and hypoglycaemia. Consequently, this can inhibit ovulation. Prolactin release is also increased during pregnancy and lactation.

Because of its role in postmenopausal breast cancer, the effect of regular physical activity on prolactin secretion has repeatedly been examined. These studies demonstrated an association between increasing physical fitness and reduced basal and stress-induced prolactin concentrations (Tworoger *et al.*, 2007). Assessment of prolactin levels during simulated marine windsurfing revealed reduced prolactin values in male world-class windsurfers (Melis *et al.*, 2003), thus indicating an increase in dopamine turnover. In contrast, marathon running and endurance training resulted in elevated prolactin levels (Daly *et al.*, 2005; Karkoulias *et al.*, 2008).

Release of hormones via the posterior pituitary

The posterior pituitary is more a collection of hypothalamic axons than a gland. Axons extend from the paraventricular nucleus and supraoptic nucleus and synthesize two peptide hormones, oxytocin and AVP. These hormones are stored in vesicles at the posterior pituitary. In response to an arriving action potential, they are secreted into the bloodstream and distributed to target cells. AVP is released in response to reductions in plasma volume (dehydration) leading to an elevation in blood pressure via vasoconstriction, and causing the kidneys to reduce urine volume, leading to a retention of water. In addition, it interacts with the HPA axis: AVP enhances the effects of CRH and thus stimulates the secretion of ACTH from the anterior pituitary.

Oxytocin (from the Greek *oxyx*, meaning 'fast' and *tokos*, meaning 'delivery') has its main effects in female reproduction by stimulating contractions of the uterus during labour and facilitating breastfeeding. Stimulation of the nipples activates the hypothalamus to secrete the 'bonding hormone' oxytocin, which, in turn, stimulates lactation due to contraction of the mammary gland. Recent data provide supportive evidence for the stimulatory effects of exercise on AVP plasma levels, depending on duration and intensity (Inder *et al.*, 1998). Furthermore, there seems to be a difference between trained and untrained individuals, with higher exercise-induced AVP values in athletes (Merry *et al.*, 2008). Only a few studies have examined oxytocin during exercise. They suggest that continuous exercise activity lasting more than 60 minutes is a potent stimulus of oxytocin secretion (Hew-Butler *et al.*, 2008).

The sympathetic adrenal–medullary system

The sympathetic adrenal–medullary system – part of the autonomic nervous system – triggers the release of catecholamines from the adrenal medulla. According to a new concept, three peripheral catecholamine systems are postulated (Goldstein, 2003): the *sympathetic nervous system* with the release of noradrenaline from sympathetic nerve terminals, the *adrenal–medullary hormonal system* with the release mainly of adrenaline, and the *DOPA–dopamine autocrine/paracrine systems* where dopamine is produced within cells, released and acts on the same or nearby cells. The author suggested that there is a difference between these three catecholamine systems depending on the stressor. This questions the notion of a unitary sympathetic adrenal–medullary system.

All three endogenous catecholamines and their metabolites can be assessed in body fluids, such as adrenaline and noradrenaline in blood and urine, or alpha-amylase and the noradrenaline metabolite 3-methoxy-4-hydroxyphenylglycolin (MHPG) in saliva. Chapters 5 and 6 present a more comprehensive review and evaluation of these analytes.

Study techniques in psychoneuroendocrinology

Where to measure hormones?

Concentration of hormones of different endocrine axes and levels can be measured in different body liquids: cerebrospinal fluid (free and bound hormones), blood (free and bound hormones), urine (free and conjugated (sulfated and glucuronidated), but not protein-bound hormones), saliva and hair (just unbound hormones).

Cerebrospinal fluid circulates around the brain and spinal cord and can be obtained by lumbar puncture in an attempt to measure levels of proteins and glucose, and to count cells. However, this procedure is very complex with the insertion of a needle into the spinal canal after local anaesthesia. Because of its complexity, the need for doctoral assistance, time-consuming aftercare (patients must remain lying down for as long as six hours afterwards), and side-effects such as headache, lumbar puncture is rarely used in non-clinical psychoneuroendocrinology research.

Another method proven to be useful is blood sampling. Blood sampling allows repeated assessment at short time intervals. However, sampling itself might cause a physiological stress response and it is not easily applicable in field research because of the need for medical assistance. Compared with blood samples, saliva sampling is non-invasive, low cost and easy to obtain, even without supervision. To avoid the hour-to-hour fluctuations seen in blood or salivary measurements, 24-hour urine collection is another sampling technique. However, because of its limited feasibility (collection might be bothersome, e.g. when not being at home) this integrative hormone measurement is not applicable for periods longer than 24 hours.

Recently, a new method of analysing cortisol and other hormones in human hair has been introduced that captures longer time periods (up to six months) depending on the length of the hair and allows the retrospective determination of cortisol secretion (Kirschbaum *et al.*, 2009). There is no ideal method for assessing hormones. Hair, urine, blood and saliva tests each have their advantages and disadvantages with regard to feasibility and applicability (Table 2.2). Because of its broad application as an easy and non-invasive method for neuroendocrine research, measuring hormones in saliva will be presented in more detail.

Measuring hormones in saliva

There are three major salivary glands (the parotid, submandibular and sublingual gland) that secrete water (99.5%) and large organic molecules including proteins, glycoproteins and lipids, small organic molecules including glucose and urea, and electrolytes (0.5%). The autonomic nervous system regulates production and secretion of 1–1.5 L saliva per day. In blood, hormones are bound (95%) and unbound (5%), but only the free, biologically active hormone fraction passes from blood into saliva via passive diffusion (steroids), active transport (peptides) or pinocytosis (whereby hormones are transported within small vesicles into the cell). The plasma/saliva ratio of hormones ranges from 10 : 1 for cortisol to 100 : 1 for testosterone and therefore requires highly sensitive assays as described below.

There are various methods for collecting saliva, either for whole samples or for specific samples, under stimulated or non-stimulated conditions. Methods for collecting non-stimulated saliva include the *draining method*, in which saliva is drained from the lower lip into a storage container by tilting the head forward, the *spitting method*, in which saliva is spat into a storage container after about a minute of accumulation within the mouth, the *suction method*, in which saliva is drawn

Table 2.2 Assessing hormones in different body fluids

	Hair	Urine	Blood	Saliva
Acute stress	–	–	+	+
Chronic stress	+	+	∘	–
Laboratory	–	∘	+	+
Field	+	+	–	+

out of the mouth, and the *swab absorbent method*, in which a cotton or polyester roll is placed in the mouth to absorb the saliva sample. In contrast, stimulated whole saliva can be stimulated by gustatory (citric acid) or mechanical stimuli (chewing).

There are many advantages of these methods:

- Collecting saliva is easy with minimal training effort and without supervision.
- It is non-invasive, making it easier to recruit participants.
- It is cost-effective.
- Hormone levels in saliva are highly correlated with serum levels.

However, there are also disadvantages:

- The collection device might influence assay results. If plastic tubes are used the researcher should bear in mind that there are different degrees of affinity for the plastic. With respect to common hormones, cortisol is less likely to bind with plastic while progesterone is more likely. Thus, the most appropriate device would be glass. However, this creates obvious disadvantages (e.g. the glass tube may break).
- Using cotton or polyester rolls may not be suitable for hormones other than cortisol because they may contain components that interfere with immunoassays (e.g. phyto-oestrogens).
- Concentrated acids within collection devices will interfere with immunoassays.
- Contamination with blood may create falsely elevated hormone levels. The saliva sample should be controlled at least visually and additional tests may be necessary, such as test strips (urinary) or salivary blood contamination assays (e.g. measuring transferrin – a protein that delivers iron in blood serum).

To summarize, the most convenient saliva collection method when measuring various hormones is to express saliva through a drinking straw into a special plastic tube. For cortisol, the use of salivettes (Sarstedt, Nümbrecht, Germany) is currently viewed as the 'gold standard' (Kirschbaum and Hellhammer, 1999). Table 2.3 provides important instruction notes for collecting saliva.

Forms of measurement

One form of measurement is the assessment of hormone levels under basal conditions to measure non-stimulated activity. In the context of basal assessment, punctual measurements are often needed in practice but have the problem that there is a large inter- and intra-individual variability due to the pulsatile and periodical secretion of hormones. This can make the clear interpretation of results difficult. Furthermore, there is no information about the reactivity and feedback function of neuroendocrine axes. It is also impossible to determine the level of

Table 2.3 Instructions for collecting saliva

Time to collection	Recommendation
Up to 30 minutes before	DO NOT brush the teeth
	DO NOT have a large meal
	DO NOT drink coffee, or drinks containing acid
	DO NOT smoke
Immediately before	Rinse the mouth with water
	Wash hands
Afterwards	Store at room temperature for up to one week
	In the refrigerator for up to 2 weeks
	In the freezer ($-20°C$) if longer storage is necessary

dysfunction that may be indicated in conspicuous basal values because a single measurement may not reflect the overall physiology.

Pharmacological tests provide an efficient solution to these disadvantages. These dynamic tests offer the opportunity to study reactivity and feedback sensitivity on multiple levels of neuroendocrine axes but are not easily applicable in field testing. Dynamic tests can essentially be divided into stimulation and suppression tests. Non-pharmacological stimulation tests to measure acute physiological, including hormonal, responses to external stimuli often include psychosocial stressors that combine unpredictable, uncontrollable and social evaluative components. In the following sections, these forms of measurement will be described in more detail.

Basal assessment

Basal hormonal tests play an important role in field research. They can be performed in a single point measurement or repeatedly at short time intervals. Due to the pulsatile secretion and therefore variability of endogenous hormone levels, multiple measurements should be preferred. One example of a multiple time point measurement is to obtain various saliva samples throughout the day to assess the circadian rhythmicity of salivary cortisol and other analytes.

Another form of basal testing is the collection of 24-hour urinary free hormone levels. These measurements indicate the total daily hormone secretion and utilization. Furthermore, this provides a stable marker of output and overcomes the dilemma of blood and saliva measurements that are susceptible to fluctuations.

There are advantages and disadvantages of each method (see also Table 2.2). As mentioned above, 24-hour urine sampling might not be feasible (e.g. when not being at home). This may lead to a lack of compliance.

Measuring hormones in hair to assess cumulative cortisol secretion over a prolonged period of time is a newly proposed method which avoids this problem. Recently, hair segment analysis was applied in athletes for the first time. Endurance athletes exhibited elevated hair cortisol levels compared to non-athletes, reflecting the cortisol response to exhaustive training in the previous months. It was noteworthy that the training intensity (number of kilometres run per week, training hours per week, number of competitions over the year) was associated with increased hair cortisol levels in a dose–response fashion (cyclists < 10 km runners < half marathon runners < triathletes < marathon runners) (Skoluda *et al.*, 2011). In contrast to blood and salivary assessments, a common feature of urine and hair methods is that information about the circadian fluctuation of hormones that might also be of clinical relevance is missing.

Dynamic testing

Since basal tests are often non-diagnostic, it is necessary to perform dynamic tests that provide information regarding the function, activity, reactivity, reserve capacity and feedback sensitivity of endocrine glands or an entire neuroendocrine axis. Pharmacological dynamic tests include suppression tests to measure hyper-activity and stimulation tests to measure hypoactivity. In the following, two tests for HPA axis activity will be presented as examples: the dexamethasone suppression test (DST) and the CRH stimulation test.

The DST is used to assess various hypercortisol states including Cushing's syndrome. Dexamethasone is a synthetic glucocorticoid based on the structure of cortisol and has the same effects as normal cortisol, including anti-inflammatory and immune suppressing effects. Because this synthetic steroid is unable to cross the blood–brain barrier, dexamethasone has its main effects on the pituitary level. It is able to interfere with feedback mechanisms of the HPA axis via negative feedback to the pituitary, thereby suppressing the release of ACTH and thus the release of cortisol from the adrenal cortex. This test of HPA axis feedback sensitivity is mainly processed as a fast overnight test. A specific amount of dexamethasone is administered orally before going to bed and serum ACTH and cortisol levels are measured the next morning. Under normal healthy conditions dexamethasone should lead to the suppression of ACTH and cortisol secretion. Non-suppression is indicative of a hypercortisolaemic state, as seen in patients with Cushing's disease.

The CRH stimulation test helps to evaluate altered CRH receptor sensitivity of the pituitary and altered feedback mechanisms. CRH stimulates corticotrophic cells of the pituitary to secrete ACTH which, in turn, stimulates cortisol secretion from the adrenals. This test is processed in the afternoon due to naturally low basal values of cortisol. After a first blood sample is drawn, CRH is administered intravenousely, and further blood samples are periodically drawn for 90–180 minutes after the CRH injection.

The combined dexamethasone/CRH test is a newer and more sensitive approach to investigate HPA axis regulation. The test requires subjects to take dexamethasone the previous night orally and to receive a CRH injection the next day. Multiple blood samples are obtained to determine ACTH and cortisol. An altered glucocorticoid feedback regulation, as seen in major depression, for example, results in an excessive ACTH and cortisol response in this test due to a lower feedback sensitivity at the level of the pituitary. In normal healthy subjects,

CRH injection should not result in an inhibition of the dexamethasone-induced cortisol suppression.

Various psychosocial stress paradigms have been designed to be used as non-pharmacological dynamic tests, mainly of HPA axis regulation. One of these widely used and well-validated psychosocial laboratory stressors is the Trier Social Stress Test (TSST; Kirschbaum *et al.*, 1993). After a 30- to 45-minute resting period, this highly standardized test consists of a 3-minute preparation period, a 5-minute speech (job interview) in front of an unknown audience and a 5-minute age-appropriate mental arithmetic task. Studies employing psychosocial stressors that combine social–evaluative threat and uncontrollability, such as the TSST, repeatedly revealed two- to threefold rises in salivary cortisol levels in over 70% of tested subjects (Kudielka *et al.*, 2007).

There are only few studies comparing endocrine responses in athletes and non-athletes during psychosocial stress induced by means of the TSST. While amateur sportsmen and untrained men did not differ, elite sportsmen exhibited lower cortisol levels after exposure to the TSST (Rimmele *et al.*, 2007, 2009; Holak, 2010). As already noted by Dickerson and Kemeny (2004), paradigms that most reliably elicit stress responses include elements of uncontrollability, unpredictability and social-evaluative threat. Recently, a group version of the TSST was introduced (von Dawans *et al.*, 2010) and shown to be an effective tool for simultaneous stress induction in multiple participants.

Biochemical assessment of hormones

Hints, confounders and test criteria

Great care must be taken in the process of hormonal assessment, including sampling, handling and analysis, to gain as much information as possible. Researchers have to check for appropriate processing of tests, to control for possible confounders, and to consider quality of testing with regard to test criteria of classical test theory. Proper sampling and handling of hormones is essential and there are guidelines that have to be obeyed: to create an adequate clinical setting, to invite participants several hours before testing depending on the test, periodic blood sampling should be performed in a sitting or lying position, a catheter should be used in order to avoid stress-induced hormonal alterations due to repeated pricking, and samples from one study should be analysed in one assay. Homogeneity of the study group and standardization of external conditions should also be ensured in order to exclude many confounders.

In hormonal testing, several confounding variables have to be considered and handled (Table 2.4). Test criteria include objectivity, reliability and validity. Biological assessment prevents manipulation of test results by individuals since it does not rely on self-report, which is subject to the effects of response bias and social desirability. Most tests show satisfactory retest reliability. Measures to increase the validity of hormonal testing include the comparison with a placebo control group, comparison with another test and the evaluation of the test's

Table 2.4 Confounding variables in hormonal testing

Variable	Handling
Age, sex, ethnicity	Equal distribution in study groups
Weight	Doses relative to weight
Sleep quantity, food intake, emotional stress, smoking, alcohol, drugs, competitive sports	Maintain constant in clinical settings
Medical disease, medical drugs, drug and alcohol abuse	Exclude from study
Individual differences	Placebo control group
Women	Control of menstrual cycle phase, use of oral contraceptives, measure oestradiol and progesterone levels

sensitivity (the proportion of actual positives that are correctly identified as such, e.g. all athletes under doping are recognized as being doped) and specifity (the proportion of actual negatives that are correctly identified as such, e.g. all undoped athletes are recognized as 'clean').

Biochemical assays

Qualitative assays measure the activity of a biochemical substance while quantitative assays measure the amount of the substance. In the following, we will give a short overview of specialized biochemical assays such as biological and immunological assays and assays that measure processes such as enzyme or receptor activity.

Biological assays are conducted either *in vivo* or *in vitro* to measure the effects of a biochemical substance on target cells. One application of these assays is their use in pharmacological studies to assess the effects and side-effects of newly developed drugs. Furthermore, these assays help to understand and investigate the function of endogenous substances such as hormones. The activity of an enzyme – its kinetics and inhibition – is measured in an enzyme assay. According to the sampling method, continuous (e.g. spectrophotometric assays) and discontinuous assays (e.g. radiometric and chromatographic assays) can be distinguished. While continuous assays determine enzyme activity (the rate of reaction after adding an enzyme to a taken sample) consecutively without further processing, discontinuous assays measure the resulting concentration of substrate and product after stopping the reaction of enzyme and biochemical substance.

Immunoassay is the term used to describe a number of methods which use the same basic principle to determine the amount of a substance. These methods use the high-specific binding of antigens to antibodies to quantify specific analytes. According to the assay, both antigen and antibody may be the substance to be detected. In addition to the need for high binding specificity, it is necessary to produce a measurable signal via the use of detectable labelling. Depending on the assay, there are various techniques of labelling. Radioimmunoassays (RIA) use weakly radioactive substances as tracers and the radioactivity is followed for the detection and quantification of the target analyte. The use of enzymes as markers is also very common. Enzyme-linked immunosorbent assays (ELISA) use enzymes that catalyse a chemical reaction, resulting in a colour reaction which can be detected photometrically. Another form of optical labelling is to assess the emission of light as a result of a chemical reaction that uses synthetic compounds and oxidized species such as peroxide (chemiluminescence immunoassay, CLIA). Fluorescence immunoassays (FIA) use fluorescein, a fluorescent molecule, to measure the analyte.

Basically, there are two types of immunoassays (Figure 2.3). In the competitive immunoassay, the unknown antigen competes with the labelled antigen to bind with antibodies. Thus, the resulting amount of labelled antigen bound to antibodies can be measured and is inversely related to the concentration of antigen in the unknown sample. The non-competitive immunoassay is also known as the 'sandwich assay'. Here the antigen is bound to the antibody and then the unoccupied binding site of the antigen is bound with labelled detector antibody. The measured amount of labelled antibody is directly proportional to the concentration of the unknown antigen.

Receptor assays use labelled enzymes that bind to specific receptors. This helps to quantify the amount of existing receptors on the cells. One application of this method is to determine whether cell growth is influenced or can be treated by hormones such as, for example, in cases of breast cancer.

Summary

In this chapter we outlined and discussed general principles of hormone release and effects as well as determination methods. Hormone levels and behaviour are interrelated – changes in hormones lead to behavioural changes and vice versa. Furthermore, hormones interact with each other. Thus, the effects of one

Competitive immunoassay   **Non-competitive immunoassay**

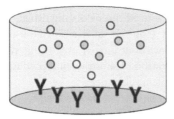   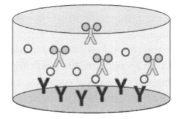

○ Target analyte   ○ Target analyte
◉ Assay conjugate labelled   Detector antibody labelled
Y Antibody   Y Antibody

Figure 2.3 Competitive and non-competitive assays for the detection of biomarkers.

hormone might be influenced by changes in levels of another hormone. Hormones often act gradually, they may have behavioural and physiological effects even hours or weeks after secretion into the bloodstream. One hormone may have multiple effects on various cells, organs and behaviour; while one behaviour or physiological response may be affected by various hormones. Hormone levels vary throughout the diurnal cycle, coordinated by 'circadian clocks' within the brain. According to their chemical structure, there are three classes of hormones: protein or peptide hormones, monoamines, and steroid hormones. Hormones affect only cells that express hormone-specific receptors (the key–lock principle) and hormonal signal transduction is classified into three classes: autocrine, paracrine and endocrine (special case: neuroendocrine) signalling.

The release of hormones via the hypothalamus, the pituitary and – in the case of trophic hormones – peripheral endocrine glands has been described, including the HPA, HPT, HPS and HPP axes. To introduce techniques in the study of psychoneuroendocrinology, we provided a discussion of where to measure hormones, different forms of measurement (basal assessment versus dynamic testing) and a short introduction to the biochemical assessment of hormones (confounders, test criteria, biochemical assays).

References

Belanoff, J. K., Gross, K., Yager, A. and Schatzberg, A. F. (2001). Corticosteroids and cognition. *Journal of Psychiatric Research*, 35, 127–145.

Bjorntorp, P. (2001). Do stress reactions cause abdominal obesity and comorbidities? *Obesity Reviews*, 2, 73–86.

Bonifazi, M., Mencarelli, M., Fedele, V., Ceccarelli, I., Pecorelli, A., Grasso, G., Aloisi, A.M. and Muscettola, M. (2009). Glucocorticoid receptor mRNA expression in peripheral blood mononuclear cells in high trained compared to low trained athletes and untrained subjects. *Journal of Endocrinological Investigation*, 32, 816–820.

Chrousos, G. P. and Gold, P. W. (1992). The concepts of stress and stress system disorders: overview of physical and behavioral homeostasis. *Journal of the American Medical Association*, 267, 1244–1252.

Ciloglu, F., Peker, I., Pehlivan, A., Karacabey, K., Ilhan, N., Saygin, O. and Ozmerdivenli, R. (2005). Exercise intensity and its effects on thyroid hormones. *Neuroendocrinology Letters*, 26, 830–834.

Daly, W., Seegers, C. A., Rubin, D. A., Dobridge, J. D. and Hackney, A. C. (2005). Relationship between stress hormones and testosterone with prolonged endurance exercise. *European Journal of Applied Physiology*, 93, 375–380.

Dickerson, S. S. and Kemeny, M. E. (2004). Acute stressors and cortisol responses: a theoretical integration and synthesis of laboratory research. *Psychological Bulletin*, 130, 355–391.

Elias, A. N. and Wilson, A. F. (1993). Exercise and gonadal function. *Human Reproduction*, 8, 1747–1761.

Frisch, H. (1999). Growth hormone and body composition in athletes. *Journal of Endocrinological Investigation*, 22, 106–109.

Ganong, W. F. (2000). Circumventricular organs: definition and role in the regulation of endocrine and autonomic function. *Clinical and Experimental Pharmacology and Physiology*, 27, 422–427.

Goldstein, D. S. (2003). Catecholamines and stress. *Endocrine Regulation*, 37, 69–80.

Hackney, A. C. (2008). Effects of endurance exercise on the reproductive system of men: the 'exercise-hypogonadal male condition'. *Journal of Endocrinological Investigation*, 31, 932–938.

Heuser, I. J., Wark, H. J., Keul, J. and Holsboer, F. (1991). Hypothalamic-pituitary-adrenal axis function in elderly endurance athletes. *Journal of Clinical Endocrinology and Metabolism*, 73, 485–488.

Hew-Butler, T., Noakes, T. D., Soldin, S. J. and Verbalis, J. G. (2008). Acute changes in endocrine and fluid balance markers during high-intensity, steady-state, and prolonged endurance running: unexpected increases in oxytocin and brain natriuretic peptide during exercise. *European Journal of Endocrinology*, 159, 729–737.

Holak, R. R. (2010). Do athletes respond differently to academic and social stress? An examination of cortisol and perceived stress throughout a semester in college athletes and typical college students. *Behavioral Neuroscience Honors Papers*. Paper 1. http://digitalcommons.conncoll.edu/bneurosciencehp/1

Holsboer, F. (2000) The corticosteroid receptor hypothesis of depression. *Neuropsychopharmacology*, 23, 477–501.

Inder, W. J., Hellemans, J., Swanney, M. P., Prickett, T. C. and Donald, R. A. (1998). Prolonged exercise increases peripheral plasma ACTH, CRH, and AVP in male athletes. *Journal of Applied Physiology*, 85, 835–841.

Karkoulias, K., Habeos, I., Charokopos, N., Tsiamita, M., Mazarakis, A., Pouli, A. and Spiropoulos, K. (2008). Hormonal responses to marathon running in non-elite athletes. *European Journal of Internal Medicine*, 19, 598–601.

Kirschbaum, C., Pirke, K. M. and Hellhammer, D. H. (1993). The Trier Social stress Test – a tool for investigating psychobiological stress responses in a laboratory setting. *Neuropsychobiology*, 28, 76–81.

Kirschbaum, C. and Hellhammer, D. H. (1999). Hypothalamus-hypophysen-nebennierenrindenachse. In D. H. Hellhammer and C. Kirschbaum (eds), *Enzyklopädie der Psychologie. Psychoendokrinologie und Psychoimmunologie, Biologische Psychologie*, Volume 3 (pp. 79–140). Göttingen: Hogrefe.

Kirschbaum, C., Tietze, A., Skoluda, N. and Dettenborn, L. (2009). Hair as a retrospective calendar of cortisol production – increased cortisol incorporation into hair in the third trimester of pregnancy. *Psychoneuroendocrinology*, 34, 332–337.

Kudielka, B. M., Hellhammer, D. H. and Kirschbaum, C. (2007). Ten years of research with the Trier Social Stress Test (TSST) revisited. In E. Harmon-Jones and P. Winkielman (eds), *Social Neuroscience: Integrating Biological and Psychological Explanations of Social Behavior* (pp. 56–83). New York: The Guilford Press.

Luger, A., Deuster, P. A., Kyle, S. B., Gallucci, W. T., Montgomery, L. C., Gold, P. W., Loriaux, D. L. and Chrousos, G. P. (1987). Acute hypothalamic-pituitary-adrenal responses to the stress of treadmill exercise. Physiologic adaptations to physical training. *New England Journal of Medicine*, 316, 1309–1315.

Mastorakos, G. and Pavlatou, M. (2005). Exercise as a stress model and the interplay between the hypothalamus-pituitary-adrenal and the hypothalamus-pituitary-thyroid axes. *Hormone and Metabolic Research*, 37, 577–584.

Mastorakos, G., Pavlatou, M., Diamanti-Kandarakis, E. and Chrousos, G. P. (2005). Exercise and the stress system. *Hormones (Athens)*, 4 (2), 73–89.

Melis, F., Crisafulli, A., Rocchitta, A., Tocco, F. and Concu, A. (2003). Does reduction of blood prolactin levels reveal the activation of central dopaminergic pathways conveying reward in top athletes? *Medical Hypotheses*, 61, 133–135.

Merry, T. L., Ainslie, P. N., Walker, R. and Cotter, J. D. (2008). Fitness alters fluid regulatory but not behavioural responses to hypohydrated exercise. *Physiology and Behavior*, 95, 348–352.

Nindl, B. C., Kraemer, W. J., Deaver, D. R., *et al.* (2001). LH secretion and testosterone concentrations are blunted after resistance exercise in men. *Journal of Applied Physiology*, 91, 1251–1258.

Pilz-Burstein, R., Ashkenazi, Y., Yaakobovitz, Y., *et al.* (2010). Hormonal response to Taekwondo fighting simulation in elite adolescent athletes. *European Journal of Applied Physiology*, 110, 1283–1290

Rimmele, U., Zellweger, B. C., Marti, B., *et al.* (2007). Trained men show lower cortisol, heart rate and psychological responses to psychosocial stress compared with untrained men. *Psychoneuroendocrinology*, 32, 627–635.

Rimmele, U., Seiler, R., Marti, B., Wirtz, P. H., Ehlert, U. and Heinrichs, M. (2009). The level of physical activity affects adrenal and cardiovascular reactivity to psychosocial stress. *Psychoneuroendocrinology*, 34, 190–198.

Rogol, A. D. (2010). Drugs of abuse and the adolescent athlete. *Italian Journal of Pediatrics*, 36, 19.

Skoluda, N., Dettenborn, L., Stalder, T. and Kirschbaum, C. (2011). Elevated hair cortisol concentrations in endurance athletes. *Psychoneuroendocrinology* (in press).

Tworoger, S. S., Sorensen, B., Chubak, J., *et al.* (2007). Effect of a 12-month randomized clinical trial of exercise on serum prolactin concentrations in postmenopausal women. *Cancer Epidemiology, Biomarkers and Prevention*, 16, 895–899.

von Dawans, B., Kirschbaum, C. and Heinrichs, M. (2010). The Trier Social Stress Test for Groups (TSST-G): A new research tool for controlled simultaneous social stress exposure in a group format. *Psychoneuroendocrinology*, 36, 514–522.

Widdowson, W. M., Healy, M. L., Sönksen, P. H. and Gibney, J. (2009). The physiology of growth hormone and sport. *Growth Hormone and IGF Research*, 19, 308–319.

Part II

Markers

Katharina Strahler and Felix Ehrlenspiel

Research into the effects of hormones in sport started to gain momentum in the early 1980s, when hormonal responses to competition were investigated (e.g. Elias, 1981). Once simpler methods for collecting and analysing samples began to be developed, more and more hormones and biomarkers of endocrine activity began to be detected. Nevertheless, today, at the beginning of the twenty-first century, psychoneuroendocrinology in sport and exercise still centres around just a few hormones. The following section will introduce them to the reader in a short and informative overview.

First, Ferran Suay presents cortisol, the 'stress hormone'. This is characterized by its rise in the morning and slow decrease throughout the day. Research on this hormone was initially stimulated by the finding that it can easily be measured in saliva samples (Kirschbaum and Hellhammer, 1994). Since then, a vast amount of studies have explored its role in stress, stress-related behaviour and health consequences. In Chapter 4, Claudia Windisch, Mirko Wegner and Henning Budde present another well-known hormone: testosterone. Recognized for its relation with aggressive behaviour and dominance (e.g. Archer, 2006), studies on testosterone and sport usually focus on sports competitions. In Chapter 5, Martin Schönfelder, Thorsten Schulz and Jana Strahler present the catecholamines adrenaline and noradrenaline. While adrenaline is at first sight tightly associated with stress or anxiety before and during competitions (e.g. Blimkie *et al.*, 1978), this chapter also highlights the catecholamines' role in metabolism. Last, but not least, in Chapter 6, Jana Strahler introduces salivary alpha-amylase, an enzyme that has recently seen rising interest in psychoneuroendocrinological research in sport and exercise and that appears to represent a general biomarker for the activity of the autonomic nervous system that can be assessed via salivary samples (Rohleder *et al.*, 2004).

Each chapter presents a summary of the physiology of each substance before considering methodological aspects. Furthermore, a short review highlights the interaction between the respective hormone or biomarker and sport behaviour, with a focus on the effects of physical and psychological stimuli on hormone activity. Thus, each part provides an overview of important aspects for starting psychoneuroendocrine research in sport and exercise.

References

Archer, J. (2006). Testosterone and human aggression: an evaluation of the challenge hypothesis. *Neuroscience and Biobehavioral Reviews*, 30, 319–345.

Blimkie, C., Cunningham, D. and Leung, F. (1978). Urinary catecholamine excretion during competition in 11 to 23 year old hockey players. *Medicine And Science in Sports*, 10, 183–193.

Elias, M. (1981). Serum cortisol, testosterone, and testosterone-binding globulin responses to competitive fighting in human males. *Aggressive Behavior*, 7, 215–224.

Kirschbaum, C. and Hellhammer, D. H. (1994). Salivary cortisol in psychoneuroendocrine research: Recent developments and applications. *Psychoneuroendocrinology*, 19, 313–333.

Rohleder, N., Nater, U. M., Wolf, J. M., Ehlert, U. and Kirschbaum, C. (2004). Psychosocial stress-induced activation of salivary alpha-amylase: An indicator of sympathetic activity? *Annals of the New York Academy of Sciences*, 1032, 258–263.

3 Cortisol

Ferran Suay and Alicia Salvador

The sympathetic adrenal–medullary (SAM) system and the hypothalamus–pituitary–adrenal (HPA) axis are the main neuroendocrine systems initiating and organizing the responses needed for the fight-or-flight reaction (Cannon, 1915). An essential feature of this fight-or-flight response is that it prepares the organism for situations demanding high energy expenditure. This stress response is triggered by the hypothalamus mainly through the sympathetic nervous system (SNS) and maintained by the activity of the above neuroendocrine systems in every situation involving physical effort. They coordinate the response of many other physiological systems to a variety of stressors, including the immune and cardiovascular systems, as well as energy production and utilization and, ultimately, also behaviour.

The SAM system activity induces a first rapid response that potentiates basic adaptations, resulting in increased perspiration and heart rate, enhanced reflexes and visual sensitivity (dilation of the pupils) or downregulation of the gastrointestinal system, among others. A second slower response is directed by the HPA axis and cortisol, its main final product, which finally helps to restore homeostasis after a stress response. In a more psychological level of analysis, high endogenous cortisol levels are generally considered to be a sign of stress and anxiety (Brown *et al.*, 1996). Together with testosterone, the end-product of the hypothalamus–pituitary–gonadal (HPG) axis, cortisol binds to steroid-responsive centres in the amygdala (Wood, 1996), a brain structure closely involved in emotional processing (LeDoux, 2000) in which both steroids exert opposing effects, with testosterone enhancing approaching behaviour (fight) and cortisol facilitating an avoiding behaviour (flight) (Schulkin, 2003). All of those responses are central in the behaviour related to exercise and sports, which usually involves physical effort and agonistic/competitive behaviour. In sports, examples of approaching behaviour may be attacks and counter-attacks in combat sports as well as in team sports such as football or handball, among other. The avoiding behaviours may involve defensive movements or positions, attempts to lose time or even faking pain or injury.

Physiology and mechanism

Cortisol synthesis

The activation of the HPA axis begins with the hypothalamic release of corticotrophin-releasing hormone (CRH) and arginine vasopressin (AVP) into the portal system. In the pituitary gland, both of these stimulate the production and secretion of adrenocorticotrophic hormone (ACTH). At the adrenal gland, ACTH acts on the common precursor of all steroid hormones, cholesterol, which is transformed into pregnenolone and – after a series of chemical reactions – into cortisol, the main human glucocorticoid mainly produced in the zona fasciculata of the adrenal gland.

Cortisol secretion and rhythmicity

As in the case of other steroid hormones, corticosteroids are produced and released at the same time. Nevertheless, variations in plasmatic concentrations of cortisol may not be interpreted solely as production shifts since some other factors are known to affect these concentrations. Among the most important, changes in plasma volume or in metabolic clearance rate should be listed in relation to sports and physical exercise, since both of them may be strongly altered by physical effort.

Under normal circumstances ACTH and cortisol secretion follows a pronounced diurnal rhythm with cortisol levels being high in the early morning (6–8 a.m.), substantially increasing (50–150%) in the 30–45 minutes after waking (cortisol awakening response, CAR), subsequently declining over the remainder of the day and falling to a nadir around midnight, or even later (Lavin, 2009). Normal secretion rates are of about 17 mg per day in the adult human male and 10% less in the female, ranging from 15–20 μg/100 mL in the morning to 1–5 μg/100 mL at midnight. Cortisol half-life is about 70–90 minutes.

Cortisol circulation

The biologically active form is free cortisol that is directly available for action, and constitutes about 1–10% of the total circulating concentrations of this hormone. The majority of cortisol (90%) is bound to and transported by the cortisol-binding globulin (CBG, also known as transcortin) or to albumin. This conjugated form acts as a reservoir to prevent acute depletion of the free cortisol fraction such as those forms produced during the night or under stress circumstances.

Metabolism of glucocorticoids occurs mostly in the liver and, to a lesser extent, in the kidneys. Once they have been inactivated, steroids are eliminated as urinary metabolites. In the case of cortisol, these metabolites are referred to as 17-hydroxycorticosteroids and their determination in 24-hour urine is used to assess the status of adrenal steroid production (Molina, 2006).

Cortisol effects

Like every other steroid, cortisol is a lipophilic hormone which enters the cell by passive diffusion and binds to the cytoplasmic glucocorticoid receptor. Then, the hormone–receptor complex enters the nucleus and exerts its physiological effects by altering transcription of genes. Since all cells express glucocorticoid receptors, the physiological effects of cortisol are brought about on almost all human tissues. Regarding exercise it has to be highlighted that cortisol affects intermediary metabolism, stimulates proteolysis and inhibits protein synthesis, increases gluconeogenesis and fatty acid mobilization (Molina, 2006) and also exerts a redistributive effect on the regulation of immune processes. The main physiological effects of cortisol are summarized in Table 3.1.

At the molecular level, glucocorticoid activity is mediated through cell-specific actions of two members of the nuclear receptor family – the glucocorticoid receptor and the mineralocorticoid receptor. Their importance for energy homeostasis is clearly highlighted by pathological states of endogenous glucocorticoid production, either by deficiency as in Addison's disease, or by an excess as in Cushing's syndrome. In Addison's disease, the resulting deficiency in proper glucocorticoid action is associated with impaired stress resistance, lymphoid tissue hypertrophy, weight loss and hypoglycaemia. In contrast, patients with Cushing's disease have sustained and pronounced hypersecretion of glucocorticoids and show a subsequent elevation of circulating glucocorticoid levels and display central obesity, increased breakdown of skeletal muscle mass, hyperglycaemia, hepatic steatosis, hypertension, elevated cholesterol, immunodeficiency and insulin resistance (Rose *et al.*, 2010)

Table 3.1 Physiological effects of glucocorticoids

System	Effects
Metabolism	Muscle protein degradation
	Nitrogen excretion
	Increased gluconeogenesis and plasmatic glycaemia
	Decreased glucose and amino acid utilization
	Increased fat utilization, fat redistribution
	Permissive effects on catecholamine and glucagon actions
Circulatory	Maintenance of vascular integrity and reactivity and fluid volume
	Maintenance of catecholamine pressor effects responsivity
Immune	Increases of anti-inflammatory cytokine production, neutrophil, platelet and red blood cell counts
	Decreases of proinflammatory cytokine production, circulating eosinophile, basophil and lymphocyte counts
	Inhibition of prostaglandin production, serotonin inflammatory effects
	Impairment of cell-mediated immunity
Central nervous system	Modulation of perception/cognition and emotion
Endocrine	Reduction of CRH and ACTH release

Metabolic effects of cortisol

As has been mentioned above, catecholamines (adrenaline and noradrenaline) released by the SAM system are the first hormonal products secreted into the bloodstream during exposure to stress. They play a central role in energy metabolism, initiating the breakdown of carbohydrates and lipids that will afterwards be sustained by the activity of glucocorticoids. In a normal sedentary state, catecholamines only account for 2–3% of 24-hour energy expenditure (Astrup, 1995).

In the peripheral tissues, cortisol acts as a catabolic hormone, inhibiting the cellular uptake of glucose to exert one of its most known effects, the rising of blood glucose levels (hyperglycaemia). This action on the carbohydrate metabolism is the origin of their denomination as glucocorticoids. But this hormone also increases the release of free amino acids and reduces protein synthesis in muscle cells. For protein degradation, it has been shown that high basal levels of cortisol do increase protein breakdown in skeletal human muscle (Gore *et al.*, 1993). This effect can be easily observed in long-distance runners and other endurance sports performers, and hypercortisolism has also been reported in female runners (Lindholm *et al.*, 1995) and male swimmers (Bonifazi *et al.*, 2009). Although cortisol is mainly known as a catabolic hormone, it also has anabolic effects on the hepatic tissue, where it increases amino acid uptake as well as the synthesis of enzymes, proteins, glucose and glycogen.

Cortisol also increases fat metabolism, thereby facilitating the lipolytic actions of catecholamines and growth hormone, which are very relevant for the energy supply during sustained physical effort, and inhibits fat production. Nevertheless, the effects of cortisol on fat tissue are complex. In spite of its lipolytic action, it is well known that cortisol secretion or production is regularly increased in obesity (Müssig *et al.*, 2010). One of the main symptoms of Cushing's syndrome, for example, is the abnormal accumulation of abdominal fat (Lonn *et al.*, 1994).

Circulatory effects of cortisol

Cortisol is essential to maintain normal vascular integrity and responsiveness as well as the volume of body fluids. It is also needed for normal renal function. Its mineralocorticoid action is responsible for the excretion of water as well as for part of normal sodium retention and potassium excretion (Kaplan, 1995).

Cortisol effects on immune activity

Glucocorticoids regulate immunity at a systemic level, while neural pathways regulate immunity at a local and regional level. Glucocorticoids play a primary role in the negative regulation of inflammatory responses and cortisol is recognized as the most potent anti-inflammatory hormone in the body (Silverman *et al.*, 2010).

Although catecholamines, CRH and beta-endorphin also play a role, glucocorticoids are the main hormonal inhibitors of immune activity. The rise of glucocorticoid blood concentrations during a stress response may halt the formation of new lymphocytes in the thymus. Cortisol inhibits the release of messengers, such as interleukins and interferons, and makes circulating lymphocytes less responsive to infection. It causes lymphocytes to be removed from the circulating blood and go back to storage in immune tissues and, moreover, may even actually kill lymphocytes. But there is also an effect of the immune system on the HPA axis. During infections, the chemical messenger interleukin-1, released by the immune system, stimulates the release of CRH in the hypothalamus, thereby activating the hormonal cascade leading to the production and secretion of cortisol by the adrenal cortex. Thus, it is as if the immune system is encouraging an endocrine effect which would ultimately suppress its own activity – a kind of self-regulatory action (Sapolsky, 2004).

Corticosteroid actions on the immune system are considered to provide a central explanation for the effects of physical exercise and training on the immune system. In essence, the immune system is enhanced during moderate and severe exercise, but intense, long-duration exercise is followed by immunodepression, which also includes suppressed natural killer cells and lymphokine-activated killer cytotoxicity and secretory IgA in the mucosa. This altered and suppressed immunity is called 'the open window', during which viruses and bacteria may gain a foothold, increasing the risk of subclinical and clinical infection (Nieman and Pedersen, 1999). The 'open window' in the immune system has been reported to last 3–72 hours, depending on the parameter measured. Endurance sports practitioners such as marathoners, triathletes and others are at an increased risk of developing upper respiratory tract infections (URTIs) following races and periods of hard training, which are associated with temporary changes in the immune system. The majority of the reported changes are decreases in function or concentration of certain immune cells. Moreover, as will be seen in Chapter 8, one reason for the overtraining impairments seen in elite athletes could be that this window of opportunism for pathogens is longer and the degree of immunosuppression more pronounced (Pedersen *et al.*, 1996).

Central nervous system effects of cortisol

Cortisol exerts its actions through binding to two types of intracellular receptors, the glucocorticoid receptor and the mineralocorticoid receptor. The glucocorticoid receptor initiates or represses gene transcription and induces negative feedback of the HPA axis through receptors on the hypothalamus and pituitary, while the mineralocorticoid receptor regulates basal activity of the HPA axis.

Scientific studies have consistently demonstrated that glucocorticoid receptor function is impaired in major depression, resulting in reduced glucocorticoid receptor-mediated negative feedback on the HPA axis and increased production and secretion of CRH in various brain regions postulated to be involved in the causality of major depression. Hyperactivity of the HPA axis is the main biochemical change, besides disturbed monoaminergic neurotransmission, observed in patients with major depression (Nikisch, 2009). Over-activity of the HPA axis has also been shown to affect sleep patterns (Antonijevic, 2008) and is liable to exert effects over other important behavioural functions such as nutrition.

Cortisol interaction with other hormones

The interactions of cortisol with other hormones are also of great interest for an understanding of energy supply during physical effort. Although there are many others, we will address the interactions of cortisol with catecholamines, testosterone and growth hormone because of their influence on supplying energy during exercise.

As has been stated, cortisol complements and enhances the actions of catecholamines on carbohydrates and fat metabolism (permissive action). During sustained physical exercise, the complementarity of these hormonal actions is very useful. During the first minutes of a physical effort (0–15 minutes approximately), adrenaline and noradrenaline blood concentrations dramatically rise (50–100%) to break down substrates to provide energy for muscular contraction. After about 15 minutes cortisol increase begins to complement catecholamine actions with its own high catabolic power. After 30 minutes, cortisol decline begins (it will return to baseline levels at about 180 minutes after the onset of the effort), but adrenaline and noradrenaline will continue rising to reach a 150–200% increase above initial values 180 minutes after the onset of exercise. All of these actions together provide the necessary hormonal stimulus to maintain the energetic processes during long-lasting effort.

Also interesting are the relationships with the anabolic steroid testosterone. While testosterone inhibits the HPA axis from functioning at the hypothalamic level by decreasing the AVP function (Hoffman *et al.*, 2010), cortisol has been shown to exert inhibitory effects on all three levels of the HPG axis. At the hypothalamus, cortisol inhibits the release of gonadotrophin-releasing hormones; at the pituitary it affects the secretion of luteinizing hormone (LH) and follicle-stimulating hormone (FSH), and at the gonads it decreases testosterone production (Kraemer and Ratamess, 2005). Moreover, cortisol antagonizes testosterone actions on target cells by occupying the steroid receptors (Molina, 2006). Together with corticosteroid effects on immune activity, the inhibitory process on the HPG axis is thought to be crucial for the stress response. Its evolutionary logic is easy to understand in terms of favouring all the organism's actions intended for immediate survival (energy supply) above the ones oriented to long-term benefits (e.g. reproduction or growth) which are triggered and maintained by testosterone.

Cortisol and growth hormone exert complementary effects on fat consumption, since blood concentrations of growth hormone begin to rise after the first 40 minutes of an aerobic effort, when cortisol is declining. Growth hormone thereby contributes to maintaining a stable supply of free fatty amino acids for the muscle cells (Wilmore *et al.*, 2008). Resting concentrations of both hormones are negatively correlated (Dinan *et al.*, 1994). This effect seems to be centrally mediated. It has been shown that abdominal obesity is related to weak glucocorticoid receptor reactivity in the hippocampus, which ultimately modifies the HPA axis responses. Nevertheless, the relationship between these two hormones is far from being completely understood (McMurray and Hackney, 2005). For example, the effects of cortisol and growth hormone on lipolysis are not totally additive when co-administered (Djurhuus *et al.*, 2002) and a normal circadian rhythm for cortisol has been reported in short-stature boys despite the abnormal growth hormone pulse amplitude (Hermida *et al.*, 1999).

Determination and assessment

Total cortisol concentrations in blood can be measured in plasma or serum, although the free fraction can also be measured in those fluids. Numerous commercial kits are available to carry out these analyses by means of radioimmunoassay (RIA) or enzyme immunoassay (ELISA; see Chapter 2). There are very wide individual differences in the cortisol levels, with normal values for a blood sample taken at 8 a.m. ranging between 6 and 23 µg/dL. In recent decades, the measurement of cortisol in saliva has become more widely accepted as a good index for plasma free cortisol and has the great advantage of being a non-invasive procedure (Kirschbaum and Hellhammer, 1994). Salivary cortisol is now accepted as a tool for physiological and diagnostic studies, being employed in screening tests for the diagnosis of several disorders such as hypercortisolism, and salivary cortisol has also been accepted as a good index of HPA axis functioning in normal subjects. A number of studies in a broad range of research have increasingly employed it in different human fields such as occupational, health or sports investigation.

As mentioned above, salivary cortisol measurement by RIA or other valid methods is an excellent index of plasma free cortisol concentration, independently of flow rate or transcortin fluctuations. In addition, samples are obtained by non-invasive stress-free procedures, are easier to collect and can obviate many problems such as the lack of skilled personnel. Saliva samples may be collected many times a day and in very different contexts; such testing can provide detailed information for physiological and diagnostic studies.

Collecting salivary samples, although easy, has several requisites that must be accomplished in order to guarantee the validity of the measurements. Many conditions exist at different levels. For instance, smoking or food intake has to be avoided in at least the 2 hours before sampling. Vigorous exercise should also be avoided in at least the 2 hours, preferably longer, before saliva is collected for measurement of cortisol if it is not the aim of the study. Information should be collected and the results statistically controlled for several conditions, such as medication, including oral contraceptives and/or alcohol/drug consumption. Usually during the sampling period, subjects are told to only drink water and to refrain from eating. They should also not take part in sports and should not brush their teeth to avoid potential blood contamination.

Because of the importance of the circadian rhythms, time of sampling is always very important and it has to be carefully recorded and included in the statistical analyses. In longitudinal designs, samples should be collected at the same time of year.

It is also important to use the same – or otherwise made comparable – laboratory techniques to compensate for any variation in results obtained by different laboratory techniques, although cross-comparisons of absolute concentrations should be avoided. The establishment of reference intervals for the population studied and method used is recommended.

For saliva collection, the direct saliva method may be employed. Saliva may be collected in sterile tubes using the passive drool method, in which subjects directly expectorate into a tube. Although it is simple, the main problem with this technique is getting enough volume. Nevertheless, for cortisol, saliva samples are often collected with devices such as the 'Salivette' (Sarstedt, Rommelsdorf, Germany). Sometimes it is suggested that additives such as citric acid should be used to increase saliva production prior to collection but since this interferes with many immunoassays, it is not recommended.

Salivary samples can be stored at room temperature for some hours, although it is best to keep the samples in the refrigerator or freezer. Most convenient is when saliva samples have been centrifuged and stored at $-20°C$ until analysed within a year; if more time is desired, it would be better to store the samples at $-80°C$.

This non-invasive type of measurement permits several samples to be obtained, either as baseline samples or in order to describe a cortisol response, or even the recovery of this response. The cortisol rise after awakening (CAR) is considered to be an indicator of basal HPA axis activity and has increasingly been employed in research (Clow et al., 2004).

There are several ways to quantify the cortisol response. A simple method is to detect the maximum value or peak of the cortisol concentration found after the event. This way of estimating the reactivity is frequently employed in sports physiology (to assess variables such as maximum lactic acid concentrations or maximum heart rate) and depends on several measurements being taken during the response at appropriate intervals.

The method more often employed, however, is calculation of the change scores or absolute difference between the pre- and postvalues (Δ value). These measurements may produce misinterpretations if the responses are related to baseline values. This problem has sometimes been solved by employing percentage changes, that is, expressing the increases as a fraction of the baseline concentration (Diedrich and Gehrke, 1992).

In recent years, the area under curve (AUC) has increasingly been employed to measure the hormonal response, especially in the case of research related to cortisol. It comprises two elements: the overall cortisol level (total area under the curve, AUC_t) as an indicator of activity level of the HPA axis and the increase of cortisol with respect to baseline value (area under the curve increase, AUC_i), as an indicator of reactivity level of the HPA axis (Pruessner et al., 2003).

Reactivity of cortisol secretion to sport and exercise

Acute or phasic reaction

ACTH blood levels are increased after 2–15 minutes of physical exercise. In less than 1 minute after that, cortisol levels rise and remain elevated, although

ACTH concentrations may stabilize after the first half hour of exercise (Viru and Viru, 2001).

With regard to the intensity, it seems that to trigger a significant response of ACTH and cortisol the exercise must reach an intensity near the individual's anaerobic threshold (Gabriel *et al.*, 1992). Further increases above this intensity do not seem to affect cortisol levels and it has been suggested that very intense anaerobic efforts may even suppress the cortisol response (Port, 1991), probably because of the inhibiting effect of high hydrogen concentrations on adrenal function. A recent study (Hill *et al.*, 2008) supports the view that moderate (60% of the maximal oxygen uptake) to high-intensity exercise (80%) provokes increases in circulating cortisol levels, which seem to be due to a combination of haemoconcentration and HPA axis stimulation. In contrast, low-intensity exercise (40%) does not result in significant increases in cortisol levels, but, after correcting for plasma volume reduction and circadian factors, low-intensity exercise actually results in a reduction in circulating cortisol levels. However, in short intense efforts, the cortisol response increases with the duration of the exercise bout (Snegovskaya and Viru, 1993).

Chronic or tonic reaction

Hormonal reactions to physical exertion involve increases in circulatory plasma catecholamines, cortisol and growth hormone. Prolonged exercise results in glycogen depletion, which induces further counter-regulatory activity of these glucostatic hormones, which are diminished by carbohydrate supplementation during the exercise (Steinacker *et al.*, 2004).

Studies conducted on animals and humans have found that training induces adrenal hypertrophy, thus enhancing the capacity to produce glucocorticoids (Goldstein and Kopin, 2008), which is considered to be an adaptive response that increases the ability to tolerate workloads. Daily strenuous exercise appears to lead to chronic ACTH hypersecretion and adrenal hyperfunction, a phenomenon observed in humans and in laboratory animals. The ability of training to increase the capacity to handle a higher workload with less pituitary–adrenal activation is one of multiple, interrelated adaptations and is proportional to the degree of physical training. Highly trained runners demonstrate attenuated responses to exercise (Moya-Albiol *et al.*, 2001a; Salvador *et al.*, 2001) and other stressors (Moya-Albiol *et al.*, 2001b), compared with untrained and mildly trained individuals, indicating that while these subjects in basal conditions are under mild hypercortisolism, during exercise their HPA axis has acquired the ability to moderate corticoid responses. Hence, the HPA axis activation induced by acute exercise is inversely proportional to the level of physical training (Mastorakos *et al.*, 2005).

Differences between trained and untrained individuals

It is well known that glucocorticoids exert many beneficial actions in exercising humans, increasing the availability of metabolic substrates for the need for energy for muscles, maintaining normal vascular integrity and responsiveness, and protecting the organism from an overreaction of the immune system in the face of exercise-induced muscle damage (Sapolsky *et al.*, 2000).

HPA axis physiology seems to be determined by previous stressful events associated with hypercortisolism. While basal cortisol and ACTH levels have been shown to be indistinguishable between runners and sedentary controls, cortisol responses to CRH were significantly increased in endurance athletes (Heuser *et al.*, 1991). The mechanisms underlying these alterations may either be a stepwise decrease in corticotrophic sensitivity to the negative feedback signal leading to a switch to positive glucocorticoid feedback, an enhanced co-secretion of ACTH secretagogues such as vasopressin, or a combination of both.

Although the hormonal profile is expected to converge toward anabolic processes at the end of an acute bout of endurance exercise, it has been shown that plasma cortisol levels remain significantly elevated almost 2 hours after the end of the exercise following a 2-hour run (Duclos *et al.*, 1997). Given the antagonistic action of glucocorticoid on muscle anabolic processes as well as their immuno-suppressive effects, it has been hypothesized that endurance-trained individuals might develop adaptive mechanisms such as decreased sensitivity to cortisol to protect muscle and other glucocorticoid-sensitive tissues against this increased postexercise cortisol secretion (Duclos *et al.*, 2003). Nevertheless, it has been reported that in endurance trained men, 24-hour cortisol secretion under non-exercising conditions is normal and similar to that of age-matched sedentary males (Duclos *et al.*, 1997).

Psychological reactivity of cortisol

Acute or phasic reaction

Similar to the reactivity to physical stress, the HPA axis reacts rapidly to psychological stressors. Accumulated evidence employing various psychosocial stressors indicates that both in blood and salivary samples, cortisol levels gradually increase within a few minutes (usually less than 10 minutes) after stimulation onset and reach peak concentrations 10–30 minutes after stress cessation. Although reliably detected in groups of healthy individuals and patients alike, the cortisol response to acute psychosocial stress shows considerable variation between individuals (Foley and Kirschbaum, 2010).

In this context, these acute reactions have mainly been related to anticipatory processes and competition-induced anxiety. Sports competitions are well known as anxiety-eliciting contexts. According to Sapolsky (2004), the three main features of an anxiogenic situation are perfectly represented in any competitive event: the participants perceive threat, the result is uncertain and the degree of control that they may exert is relative. The competitive response of cortisol is certainly affected by the physical effort developed (Suay *et al.*, 1999). Nevertheless, the cortisol response may be initiated before the onset of any physical exertion (Salvador *et al.*, 2003), thereby revealing the psychogenic nature of its triggering. Although it could be argued that the anticipatory rises are a good preparation for the incoming physical demands, it has been shown that rises are greater before a competition than before a non-physical situation (Salvador *et al.*, 2003) or even a non-competitive physical effort involving a similar lactate change (Suay *et al.*, 1999), showing the greater ability of competition to induce cortisol rises.

In non-sports contexts cortisol has also been frequently related to anxiety (Silverman *et al.*, 2010). In humans, social interactions (Heinrichs and Gaab, 2007), competitive situations (Salvador, 2005; Salvador and Costa, 2009), maternal separation (Gunnar *et al.*, 2009), examinations (Al-Ayadhi, 2005) and many other different types of anxiogenic situations have been found to increase salivary cortisol concentrations. For another type of anxiety disorder – posttraumatic stress disorder – there is also considerable evidence for an HPA axis dysregulation consisting of enhanced feedback inhibition, as well as the suggestion that this system may play an important role in its pathophysiology (Yehuda, 2002).

Chronic or tonic reaction

In sports contexts, depression is known to be one of the most prevalent symptoms of overtraining states, as addressed in Chapter 10. It now seems clear that HPA axis dysregulation may play an important role in the pathophysiology of depression (Young *et al.*, 2003) and sustained high levels of cortisol are considered to be a possible sign of depressive disorder. The dexamethasone suppression test has been proposed as an indicator of depressive states. This test consists of injecting a high dose of dexamethasone, a synthetic corticoid that imitates the physiological actions of cortisol, and measuring the subsequent levels of cortisol. While in healthy individuals dexamethasone injection induces a rapid decrease of cortisol secretion, because of the negative feedback mechanisms of the HPA axis, in patients with major depressive disorders the test has revealed abnormal escape from suppression (Carroll *et al.*, 1981). This has been interpreted as a central overdrive of the HPA axis and impairment of its negative feedback mechanisms, mostly due to the downregulation of the hippocampal glucocorticoid receptors (Ströhle and Holsboer, 2003).

Current research

The possibility of determining cortisol levels by means of a non-invasive method such as saliva sampling has – without doubt – contributed to increasing the number of research topics studied with the aid of cortisol measures. In the sports and physical exercise field, one important focus for cortisol-centred research is related to training control and overtraining syndrome, as addressed in Chapter 10. Other than that, some particularly interesting topics referring to health-related behaviours that may be of some interest for sport psychologists will be briefly addressed here.

Stress management

As everyone has to cope with stressful situations in certain areas of life, stress management has become an important focus for scientific research, and cortisol – being considered a biological marker of stress – has been used to assess the impact of various stress-reducing strategies. Since the impact of physical exercise on cortisol levels has already been addressed above, we will focus on some exercise-like strategies which, although they are not strictly sports, may have some common points with training.

Since a sedentary lifestyle is considered a main risk factor for health, promoting active lifestyles based on a regular practice of exercise has become a main goal for governments in many countries. This goal has proved to be a difficult one and partly related to the aversive characteristics of vigorous exercise (Dishman and Buckworth, 1997). Because it has been demonstrated that regular physical exertion can exert positive effects on mental health even when it does not enhance physical condition (Dishman *et al.*, 1988), promoting an active lifestyle does not necessarily mean trying to get people involved in training practices such as vigorous running, swimming or cycling. Instead of this, the focus may switch from the promotion of sport activities to the encouragement of healthy physical leisure activities, such as walking or gardening. Such physical activities performed with no competitive or physical conditioning aims may also be considered as stress-reducing strategies. Moreover, since they are not highly demanding and not necessarily fatiguing, it may be thought that there is more chance that people will keep doing them.

Although cortisol levels have been mostly assessed in training settings, some studies have focused on low-demand activities. It has been found that – as previously commented – low-intensity exercise (40% of the Vo_{2max}) results in a reduction in circulating cortisol levels (Hill *et al.*, 2008), which allows us to consider these kinds of activities as being stress-reducing.

Again in the field of low-demanding physical activities, some studies – mostly centred on adults with medical conditions – have found decreased cortisol levels following mindfulness-based stress reduction programmes, such as yoga, tai chi or qi training (e.g. Carlson *et al.*, 2004). The cortisol decreases have been interpreted as indicators of a stress-reduction effect produced by those treatments (Carlson *et al.*, 2004, 2007; Bertisch *et al.*, 2009). However, not all studies have found decreases in cortisol levels following these practices, and it has been reported that some stress-reduction activities, such as yoga practice (Kiecolt-Glaser *et al.*, 2010), can elicit similar positive psychological effects without concomitant physiological effects, which suggests that cortisol reductions are not the only mechanism involved in the production of positive psychological effects (Matousek *et al.*, 2010).

Obesity

Obesity has also been repeatedly addressed in the area of health-related behaviour. Its prevalence has been increasing steadily in the industrialized world in recent decades and now obesity has developed into a world-wide epidemic associated with large economic costs and prevalent diseases (Barness *et al.*, 2007). The knowledge that obesity is a prominent feature of hypercortisolism (as in Cushing's syndrome) has stimulated investigation into the possibility that hypercortisolism is a feature of obesity. Hypercortisolism can exist in two forms: systemic hypercortisolism, in which there is an overall bodily excess of cortisol, and tissue hypercortisolism, in which there is increased intracellular concentration of cortisol without an overall bodily excess (Salehi *et al.*, 2005). In recent studies, cortisol has been found to be associated with the pathogenesis of obesity (Reynolds, 2010) and is now known to be involved in the maintenance of high levels of adiposity. Cortisol levels have also been used for the diagnosis of metabolic syndrome (Gade *et al.*, 2010).

Although it is well known that cortisol secretion or production is regularly increased in obesity, the reasons are only partially understood and three main potential explanations have been proposed for the observed rise in cortisol secretion: (1) it is appropriate to the increase in lean body mass in obesity; (2) it is due to an overactivity of the HPA axis; and (3) it may result from enhanced cortisol metabolic rate with compensatory changes in the HPA axis (Müssig *et al.*, 2010). Nevertheless, the majority of studies do not support the existence of systemic hypercortisolism in animal or human obesity despite frequently increased glucocorticoid secretion and excretion rates. Instead of this explanation, a growing body of evidence supports the idea that an increased enzyme activity may be the underlying pathophysiological cause of a tissue-specific intracellular cortisol excess in obesity (Müssig *et al.*, 2010).

Dominance

Dominance and submissiveness are important topics in hormone-centred research in animals (Chichinadze and Chichinadze, 2008) as well as in humans (Archer, 2006), and has also been addressed in sports settings (Salvador *et al.*, 1999). Traditionally, it is said that testosterone should increase dominance and other status-seeking behaviours (Mazur and Booth, 1998). However, empirical results have been inconsistent and there is some support for the claim that the neuroendocrine reproductive (HPG) and stress (HPA) axes interact to regulate dominance. A recent study (Mehta and Josephs, 2010) suggests that since dominance is related to stressful activities such as gaining and maintaining high status positions in social hierarchies, it is only when cortisol is low that higher testosterone levels encourage higher status. In contrast, when cortisol is high, higher testosterone may actually decrease dominance and in turn motivate lower status. This is an interesting issue in sports-related research, since dominant or submissive tendencies may be significant and important to understand in many sports contexts. In particular they are important in clarifying leadership in team sports and also in groups of individual sports practitioners, since participants are likely to be exposed to elevated cortisol levels because of their training demands.

Individual differences

The high inter-individual variability of hormonal levels is an important issue in hormonal research (Viru, 1992). It seriously prevents direct comparisons among individuals and makes it necessary to use different strategies such as percentage changes in order to compare the responses and/or adaptations of different subjects.

A key feature of salivary cortisol levels is the large variation in the response magnitude between individuals as well as – in a single subject – across different situations. Such variability can be observed in cortisol concentrations as well as in the time pattern of hormone secretion after exposure to stress.

Summary

Overall, the identification of mechanisms that determine the regulation and especially dysregulation of free cortisol responses to stress is, particularly in humans, a challenging task (Kudielka *et al.*, 2009). For that reason, researchers and also applied sport scientists willing to add cortisol determinations to their professional activities need to be aware of the multiple moderating and intervening variables that affect cortisol responses to different kinds of stressors and stimuli, in order to correctly interpret the results obtained. Since a thorough exposition of this knowledge would exceed the remit of the present chapter, we recommend the cited paper from Kudielka *et al.* (2009). Considered together with other hormonal and non-hormonal (psychological, performance, etc.) variables, cortisol measures may afford useful information for sports scientists and practitioners.

References

Al-Ayadhi, L. Y. (2005). Neurohormonal changes in medical students during academic stress. *Annals of Saudi Medicine*, 25, 36–40.

Antonijevic, I. (2008). HPA axis and sleep: identifying subtypes of major depression. *Stress*, 11, 15–27.

Archer, J. (2006). Testosterone and human aggression: an evaluation of the challenge hypothesis. *Neuroscience and Biobehavioral Reviews*, 30, 319–345.

Astrup, A. (1995). The sympathetic nervous system as a target for intervention in obesity. *International Journal of Obesity and Related Metabolic Disorders*, 19 (Suppl 7), S24–S28.

Barness, L. A., Opitz, J. M. and Gilbert-Barness, E. (2007). Obesity: genetic, molecular, and environmental aspects. *American Journal of Medical Genetics*, 143A, 3016–3034.

Bertisch, S. M., Wee, C. C., Phillips, R. S. and McCarthy, E. P. (2009). Alternative mind-body therapies used by adults with medical conditions. *Journal of Psychosomatic Research*, 66, 511–519.

Bonifazi, M., Mencarelli, M., Fedele, V., *et al.* (2009). Glucocorticoid receptor mRNA expression in peripheral blood mononuclear cells in high trained compared to low trained athletes and untrained subjects. *Journal of Endocrinological Investigation*, 32, 816–820.

Brown, L. L., Tomarken, A. J., Orth, D. N., Loosen, P. T., Kalin, N. H. and Davidson, R. J. (1996). Individual differences in repressive-defensiveness predict basal salivary cortisol levels. *Journal of Personality and Social Psychology*, 70, 362–371.

Cannon, W. B. (1915). *Bodily Changes in Pain, Hunger, Fear and Rage: An account of recent researches into the function of emotional excitement*. New York: Appleton.

Carlson, L. E., Speca, M., Patel, K. D. and Goodey, E. (2004). Mindfulness-based stress reduction in relation to quality of life, mood, symptoms of stress and levels of cortisol, dehydroepiandrosterone sulfate (DHEAS) and melatonin in breast and prostate cancer outpatients. *Psychoneuroendocrinology*, 29, 448–474.

Carlson, L. E., Speca, M., Faris, P. and Patel, K. D. (2007). One year pre-post intervention follow-up of psychological, immune, endocrine and blood pressure outcomes of mindfulness-based stress reduction (MBSR) in breast and prostate cancer outpatients. *Brain, Behaviour, and Immunity*, 21, 1038–1049.

Carroll, B.J., Feinberg, M., Greden, J.F., *et al.* (1981). A specific laboratory test for the diagnosis of melancholia. Standardization, validation, and clinical utility. *Archives of General Psychiatry*, 38, 15–22.

Chichinadze, K. and Chichinadze, N. (2008). Stress-induced increase of testosterone: contributions of social status and sympathetic reactivity. *Physiology and Behavior*, 94, 595–603.

Clow, A., Thorn, L., Evans, P. and Hucklebridge, F. (2004). The awakening cortisol response: methodological issues and significance. *Stress*, 7, 29–37.

Diedrich, O. and Gehrke, J. (1992). How to define an endocrine response. In C. Kirschbaum, G. F. Read and D. H. Hellhammer (eds), *Assessment of Hormones and Drugs in Saliva in Biobehavioral Research* (pp. 59–64). Seattle, WA: Hogrefe and Huber Publ.

Dinan, T. G., Thakore, J. and O'Keane, V. (1994). Lowering cortisol enhances growth hormone response to growth hormone releasing hormone in healthy subjects. *Acta Physiologica Scandinavica*, 151, 413–416.

Dishman, R. K. and Buckworth, J. (1997). Adherence to physical activity. Physical activity and mental health. In W. P. Morgan (ed.), *Physical Activity and Mental Health* (pp. 63–80). Philadelphia, PA: Taylor and Francis.

Dishman, R. K., Armstrong, R. B., Delp, M. D., Graham, R. E. and Dunn, A. L. (1988). Open-field behavior is not related to treadmill performance in exercising rats. *Physiology and Behavior*, 43, 541–546.

Djurhuus, C. B., Gravholt, C. H., Nielsen, S., *et al.* (2002). Effects of cortisol on lipolysis and regional interstitial glycerol levels in humans. *American Journal of Physiology Endocrinology and Metabolism*, E283, 172–177.

Duclos, M., Corcuff, J. B., Rashedi, M., Fougere, V. and Manier, G. (1997). Trained versus untrained: different hypothalamo-pituitary adrenal axis responses to exercise recovery. *European Journal of Applied Physiology*, 75, 343–350.

Duclos, M., Gouarne, C. and Bonnemaison, D. (2003). Acute and chronic effects of exercise on tissue sensitivity to glucocorticoids. *Journal of Applied Physiology*, 94, 869–875.

Foley, P. and Kirschbaum, C. (2010). Human hypothalamus-pituitary-adrenal axis responses to acute psychosocial stress in laboratory settings. *Neuroscience and Biobehavioral Reviews*, 35, 91–96.

Gabriel, H., Schwarz, L., Steffens, G. and Kindermann, W. (1992). Immunoregulatory hormones, circulating leucocyte and lymphocyte subpopulations before and after endurance exercise of different intensities. *International Journal of Sports Medicine*, 13, 359–366.

Gade, W., Schmit, J., Collins, M. and Gade, J. (2010). Beyond obesity: the diagnosis and pathophysiology of metabolic syndrome. *Annals of Clinical and Laboratory Science*, 23, 51–61.

Goldstein, D. S. and Kopin, I. J. (2008). Adrenomedullary, adrenocortical, and sympathoneural responses to stressors: a meta-analysis. *Endocrine Regulations*, 42, 111–119.

Gore, D. C., Jahoor, F., Wolfe, R. R. and Herndon, D. N. (1993). Acute response of human muscle to catabolic hormones. *Annals of Surgery*, 218, 679–684.

Gunnar, M.R., Talge, N.M. and Herrera, A. (2009). Stressor paradigms in developmental studies: what does and does not work to produce mean increases in salivary cortisol. *Psychoneuroendocrinology*, 34, 953–967.

Heinrichs, M. and Gaab, J. (2007). Neuroendocrine mechanisms of stress and social interaction: implications for mental disorders. *Current Opinion in Psychiatry*. 20, 158–162.

Hermida, R. C., García, L., Ayala, D. E. and Fernández, J. R. (1999). Circadian variation of plasma cortisol in prepubertal children with normal stature, short stature and growth hormone deficiency. *Clinical Endocrinology*, 50, 473–479.

Heuser, I. J., Wark, H. J., Keul, J. and Holsboer, F. (1991). Hypothalamic-pituitary-adrenal axis function in elderly endurance athletes. *Journal of Clinical Endocrinology and Metabolism*, 73, 485–458.

Hill, E. E., Zack, E., Battaglini, C., Viru, M., Viru, A. and Hackney, A. C. (2008). Exercise and circulating cortisol levels: the intensity threshold effect. *Journal of Endocrinological Investigation*, 31, 587–591.

Hoffman, J. R., Ratamess, N. A., Kang, J., *et al.* (2010). Examination of the efficacy of acute L-alanyl-L-glutamine ingestion during hydration stress in endurance exercise. *Journal of the International Society of Sports Nutrition*, 3, 7–8.

Kaplan, N. M. (1995). The adrenal glands. In J. E. Griffin and S. R. Ojeda (eds), *Textbook of Endocrine Physiology*, 3rd edn (pp. 284–313). New York: Oxford University Press.

Kiecolt-Glaser, J. K., Christian, L., Preston, H., *et al.* (2010). Stress, inflammation, and yoga practice. *Psychosomatic Medicine*, 72, 113–121.

Kirschbaum, C. and Hellhammer, D. H. (1994). Salivary cortisol in psychoneuroendocrine research: recent developments and applications. *Psychoneuroendocrinology*, 19, 313–333.

Kraemer, W. J. and Ratamess, N. A. (2005). Hormonal responses and adaptations to resistance exercise and training. *Sports Medicine*, 35, 339–361.

Kudielka, B. M., Hellhammer, D. H. and Wüst, S. (2009). Why do we respond so differently? Reviewing determinants of human salivary cortisol responses to challenge. *Psychoneuroendocrinology*, 34, 2–18.

Lavin, N. (2009). *Manual of Endocrinology and Metabolism*, 4th edn. Philadelphia: Lippincott Williams and Wilkins.

LeDoux, J. E. (2000). Emotion circuits in the brain. *Annual Review of Neuroscience*, 23, 155–184.

Lindholm, C., Hirschberg, A. L., Carlström, K. and von Schoultz, B. (1995). Altered adrenal steroid metabolism underlying hypercortisolism in female endurance athletes. *Fertility and Sterility*, 63, 1190–1194.

Lonn, L., Kvist, H., Ernest, I. and Sjostrom, L. (1994). Changes in body composition and adipose tissue distribution after treatment of women with Cushing's syndrome. *Metabolism*, 43, 1517–1522.

Mastorakos, G., Pavlatou, M., Diamanti-Kandarakis, E. and Chrousos, G. P. (2005). Exercise and the stress system. *Hormones*, 4(2), 73–89.

Matousek, R. H., Dobkin, P. L. and Pruessner, J. (2010). Cortisol as a marker for improvement in mindfulness-based stress reduction. *Complementary Therapies in Clinical Practice*, 16, 13–19.

Mazur, A. and Booth, A. (1998). Testosterone and dominance in men. *Behavioral and Brain Sciences*, 21, 353–363; discussion 363–397.

McMurray, R. G. and Hackney, A. C. (2005). Interactions of metabolic hormones, adipose tissue and exercise. *Sports Medicine*, 35, 393–412.

Mehta, P. H. and Josephs, R. A. (2010). Testosterone and cortisol jointly regulate dominance: evidence for a dual-hormone hypothesis. *Hormones and Behavior*, 58, 898–906.

Molina, P. E. (2006). *Endocrine Physiology*. New York: Lange Medical Books/McGraw-Hill.

Moya-Albiol, L., Salvador, A., Costa, R., *et al.* (2001a). Psychophysiological responses to the Stroop task after a maximal cycle ergometry in elite sportsmen and physically active subjects. *International Journal of Psychophysiology*, 40, 47–59.

Moya-Albiol, L., Salvador, A., González-Bono, E., Martínez-Sanchís, S. and Costa, R. (2001b). The impact of exercise on hormones is related to autonomic reactivity to a mental task. *International Journal of Stress Management*, 8, 215–229.

Müssig, K., Remer, T. and Maser-Gluth, C. (2010). Brief review: glucocorticoid excretion in obesity. *Journal of Steroid Biochemistry and Molecular Biology*, 121, 589–593.

Nieman, D.C. and Pedersen, B.K. (1999). Exercise and immune function. Recent developments. *Sports Medicine*, 27, 73–80.

Nikisch, G. (2009). Involvement and role of antidepressant drugs of the hypothalamic-pituitary-adrenal axis and glucocorticoid receptor function. *Neuroendocrinology Letters*, 30, 11–16.

Pedersen, B.K., Rohde, T. and Zacho, M. (1996). Immunity in athletes. *Journal of Sports Medicine and Physical Fitness*, 36, 236-245.

Port, K. (1991). Serum and saliva cortisol responses and blood lactate accumulation during incremental exercise testing. *International Journal of Sports Medicine*, 12, 490–494.

Pruessner, J. C., Kirschbaum, C., Meinlschmid, G. and Hellhammer, D. H. (2003). Two formulas for computation of the area under the curve represent measures of total hormone concentration versus time-dependent change. *Psychoneuroendocrinology*, 28, 916–931.

Reynolds, R. M. (2010). Corticosteroid-mediated programming and the pathogenesis of obesity and diabetes. *Journal of Steroid Biochemistry and Molecular Biology*, 122, 3–9.

Rose, A.J., Vegiopoulos, A., and Herzig, S. (2010). Role of glucocorticoids and the glucocorticoid receptor in metabolism: insights from genetic manipulations. *Journal of Steroid Biochemistry and Molecular Biology*, 122, 10–20.

Rosmond, R., Chagnon, Y. C., Holm, G., *et al.* (2000). A glucocorticoid receptor gene marker is associated with abdominal obesity, leptin, and dysregulation of the hypothalamic-pituitary-adrenal axis. *Obesity Research*, 8, 211–218.

Salehi, M., Ferenczi, A. and Zumoff, B. (2005). Obesity and cortisol status. *Hormone and Metabolic Research*, 37, 193–197.

Salvador, A. (2005). Coping with competitive situations in humans. *Neuroscience and Biobehavioral Reviews*, 29, 195–205.

Salvador, A. and Costa, R. (2009). Coping with competition: neuroendocrine responses and cognitive variables. *Neuroscience and Biobehavioral Reviews*, 33, 160–170.

Salvador, A., Suay, F., Martinez-Sanchis, S., Simon, V. M. and Brain, P. F. (1999). Correlating testosterone and fighting in male participants in judo contests. *Physiology and Behavior*, 68, 205–209.

Salvador, A., Ricarte, J., González-Bono, E. and Moya-Albiol, L. (2001). Effects of physical training on endocrine and autonomic responsiveness to acute stress. *Journal of Psychophysiology*, 15, 114–121.

Salvador, A., Suay, F., González-Bono, E. and Serrano, M. A. (2003). Anticipatory cortisol, testosterone and psychological responses to judo competition in young men. *Psychoneuroendocrinology*, 28, 364–375.

Sapolsky, R.M. (2004). *Why Zebras Don't Get Ulcers*, 3rd edn. New York: Henry Holt and Co.

Sapolsky, R. M., Romero, M. and Munck, A. U. (2000). How do glucocorticoids influence stress responses? Integrating permissive, suppressive, stimulatory, and preparative actions. *Endocrine Reviews*, 21, 55–89.

Schulkin, J. (2003). Allostasis: a neural behavioral perspective. *Hormones and Behavior*, 43, 21–27; discussion 28–30

Silverman, M. N., Heim, C. M., Nater, U. M., Marques, A. H. and Sternberg, E. M. (2010). Neuroendocrine and immune contributors to fatigue. *PM&R*, 2, 338–346.

Snegovskaya, V. and Viru, A. (1993). Elevation of cortisol and growth hormone levels in the course of further improvement of performance capacity in trained rowers. *International Journal of Sports Medicine*, 14, 202–206.

Steinacker, J. M., Lormes, W., Reissnecker, S. and Liu, Y. (2004). New aspects of the hormone and cytokine response to training. *European Journal of Applied Physiology*, 91, 382–391.

Ströhle, A. and Holsboer, F. (2003). Stress responsive neurohormones in depression and anxiety. *Pharmacopsychiatry*, 36(Suppl. 3), 207–214.

Suay, F., Salvador, A., González-Bono, E., *et al.* (1999). Effects of competition and its outcome on serum testosterone, cortisol and prolactin. *Psychoneuroendocrinology*, 24, 551–556.

Viru, A. (1992). Plasma hormones and physical exercise. *International Journal of Sports Medicine*, 13, 201–209.

Viru, A. and Viru, M. (2001). *Biochemical Monitoring of Sport Training*. Champaign, IL: Human Kinetics.

Wilmore, J. H., Costill, D. L. and Kenney, W. L. (2008). *Physiology of Sport and Exercise*, 4th edn. Champaign, IL: Human Kinetics.

Wood, R. I. (1996). Functions of the steroid-responsive neural network in the control of male hamster sexual behavior. *Trends in Endocrinology and Metabolism*, 7, 338–344.

Yehuda, R. (2002). Current status of cortisol findings in post-traumatic stress disorder. *Psychiatric Clinics of North America*, 25, 341–368.

Young, E.A., Lopez, J.F., Murphy-Weinberg, V., Watson, S.J. and Akil, H. (2003). Mineralocorticoid receptor function in major depression. *Archives of Genetical Psychiatry*, 60, 24–28.

4 Testosterone

Claudia Windisch, Mirko Wegner
and Henning Budde

The umbrella term for male sex hormones is 'androgens'; these have anabolic (protein synthesizing) effects as well as androgenic (virilizing) effects. The principal androgen is testosterone. Alongside oestrogen, it is the final product of the hypothalamic–pituitary–gonadal (HPG) axis. Endogenous stimuli such as biological rhythms or the hormones themselves, as well as external stimuli, activate the HPG axis. External stimuli include physical exercise and other forms of stress (mental, psychosocial), and they have a prolonged effect on androgen levels. Because the HPG axis interacts extensively with the hypothalamic–pituitary–adrenal (HPA) axis, somewhat similar to cortisol, testosterone increases after acute exercise once a specific intensity threshold is reached.

This chapter summarizes previous research showing that the concentration of testosterone, which can be obtained in saliva, serum and urine, influences physical and psychological variables and vice versa. Besides the acute effects, findings about long-term training interventions provide additional information that is important in sport.

Physiology and mechanisms

Biosynthesis

In humans, testosterone is primarily secreted from the Leydig cells of the testes of males, which produce between 5 and 10 mg/day. Although the ovaries of females produce high concentrations of androgens as well, high local concentrations of aromatizing enzymes rapidly convert the majority of those androgens to oestrogens before they can enter the general circulation. Small amounts of testosterone (approx. 5%) are also secreted by the adrenal cortex. Thus, total testosterone serum levels of approximately 30–60 ng/dL are found in women in comparison to 300–1200 ng/dL testosterone in male serum (Swerdloff *et al.*, 2009).

The major steps of the principal pathway of testosterone biosynthesis in humans and its most important precursors are as follows: cholesterol → pregnenolone → 17α-hydroxypregnenolone → dehydroepiandrosterone (DHEA) → androstendione → testosterone (→ 5α-dihydrotestosterone).

The most important metabolite of testosterone and its hormonally more active form is 5α-dihydrotestosterone (DHT). The reduction of testosterone to DHT occurs in those tissues expressing 5α-reductase (e.g. in prostate tissue). The plasma elimination half-life of testosterone is very short, in the range of 10–15 minutes (e.g. Lang and Verrey, 2007). Plasma elimination half-life is dependent on sex hormone-binding globulin (SHBG) concentrations, with increased SHBG levels leading to a longer half-life of testosterone (Diamanti-Kandarakis, 1999). In the liver, testosterone is degraded to 17-keto steroids (biologically inactive compounds) which are in turn conjugated to water-soluble sulfates amenable to urinary excretion.

Pathways and regulation

The regulation of testosterone release is controlled by the HPG axis. Figure 4.1 shows the underlying mechanism. In a first step, the hypothalamus, in pulsatile secretion, delivers the gonadotrophin-releasing hormone (GnRH). This reaches the anterior pituitary via the hypophyseal portal system that links the hypothalamus and the pituitary and causes the secretion of gonadotrophins such as luteinizing hormone (LH) and follicle-stimulating hormone (FSH). In turn, the released LH activates the gonads to synthesize oestrogen and testosterone (Figure 4.1). The steroid hormones testosterone (and oestrogen) give feedback to both the anterior pituitary and the hypothalamus in order to inhibit activity. In parallel,

HPG Axis

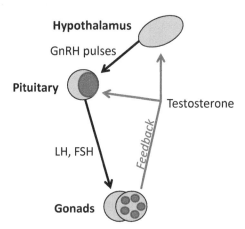

Figure 4.1 Gonadotrophin-releasing hormone (GnRH) pulses from the hypothalamus stimulate the pituitary to secrete luteinizing hormone (LH) and follicle-stimulating hormone (FSH) pulses that act on the gonads to stimulate sex steroid release (testosterone), which feed back to regulate the hypothalamus and pituitary.

increasing levels of LH and FSH slow down the gonadotrophin secretion from the anterior pituitary and GnRH secretion from the hypothalamus. Likewise, as GnRH is secreted, the hypothalamus responds to increasing levels of the hormone by slowing down its secretion.

GnRH release varies according to stage of life. For example, the negative feedback sensitivity of the hypothalamus and pituitary to circulating steroids lessens during puberty. This process is responsible for the increasing testosterone concentrations at that age.

Testosterone becomes effective through two main mechanisms: (1) by activation of the androgen receptor and (2) by aromatization to oestradiol and activation of certain oestrogen receptors. Free testosterone or DHT is transported into the cytoplasm of target tissue cells where it can bind to the androgen receptor. The testosterone–receptor complex undergoes a structural change that allows it to move into the cell nucleus. There it binds directly to specific nucleotide sequences of the chromosomal DNA, which triggers transcriptional activity of certain genes leading to the subsequent protein biosynthesis.

Through small changes in the molecular structure, the anabolic effects of the androgens increase while at the same time the androgenic effects decrease. Such anabolic steroids are used in the medical treatment of patients (e.g. after operations, in weakness, malnutrition, etc.). However, they are also abused in sports as doping substances because of their ability to promote muscle growth and further anabolic effects.

Transport and circadian rhythms

Under physiological conditions approximately 45–70% of the circulating testosterone in plasma is bound to SHBG, 30–55% to albumin with weaker bonding and approximately 2% remains in the unbound or free form. The combination of the free and the albumin-bound fraction is called the 'bioavailable testosterone'. The free fraction is biologically the most available one which can enter cells. The free diffusion of the unbound testosterone is demonstrated by the same free testosterone concentration in all body fluids, like blood and saliva. Free and protein-bound testosterone as well as DHT (which is also bound to SHBG) are in equilibrium. Thus when free hormone is subtracted from the circulation because of entry into tissue, new testosterone dissociates from albumin and SHBG in order to keep the free testosterone concentration constant (see Simoni, 2004).

Like other hormones, such as cortisol (see Chapter 3), testosterone secretion undergoes a diurnal variation with higher circulating levels observed in the early morning and decreasing levels through the rest of the daytime (see Figure 4.2, solid line).

Individual differences in testosterone production throughout the day are likely to be influenced by predispositions as well as events experienced (e.g. exercise). Both the diurnal pattern as well as the total amount of testosterone is markedly lower in elderly men than in adolescent and younger men (Diver *et al.*, 2003). As shown in Figure 4.2, there are also seasonal variations of testosterone levels

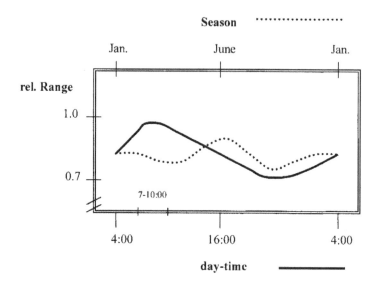

Figure 4.2 Pattern of relative changes in serum testosterone levels due to diurnal (solid line) and seasonal (dotted line) variations of testosterone secretion (data for seasonal variations apply to people living in the northern hemisphere). From Zitzmann and Nieschlag (2001). Testosterone levels in healthy men and the relation to behavioural and physical characteristics: facts and constructs. *European Journal of Endocrinology*, 144, 183–197. (c) Society of the European Journal of Endocrinology (2001). Reproduced by permission.

with a peak in the summer months (dotted line). It is especially important to note this in comparative analyses or samples from different daytimes or months, or for longitudinal study designs.

Testosterone determination

In clinical settings, the measurement of testosterone is well established for the diagnosis of hypogonadism in men or pathological androgen excess in women. Testosterone measurement also shows an association with various diseases and conditions, such as metabolic syndrome, diabetes, cardiovascular disease and neurodegenerative disorders (Vesper and Cook Botelho, 2010). In recent years, the measurement of hormones has become of particular interest for behavioural scientists testing biosocial models of individual differences and intra-individual changes in mood, cognition, behaviour and psychopathology. In the following section we summarize some useful implications and recommendations.

Because of the strong diurnal variation with morning concentrations being approximately 20–30% higher than evening values, testosterone samples should be taken during the morning hours. Only then will single point samples be representative. More sample time points are needed to obtain information about the diurnal course of testosterone or measuring testosterone concentrations in response to a stressor (e.g. exercise; Papacosta and Nassis, 2011). With regard to the time frame, immediate and 5 minutes postexercise results showed an increase in testosterone levels both in men and women (Zitzmann, 2011). Two hours after the training sessions the mean testosterone concentration returned to the pre-exercise level (Jensen *et al.*, 1991).

An economic method to obtain basal testosterone is to repeatedly sample at two or three time points before starting the intervention and calculate a mean value. So, a possible sample schedule for an acute intervention could be 30 minutes before a stressor, immediately before and immediately after a stressor, followed by three further samples after the stressor (e.g. 15, 30 and 60 minutes). Tremblay and co-workers (2005) indicate that at a low intensity, longer exercise durations are necessary to stimulate increased testosterone levels.

In order to minimize intra-individual differences, we recommend taking samples on two consecutive days at the same time points, calculating the statistical mean of these two obtained testosterone values. Measuring samples in duplicate is also a good standard procedure. The obtained intra-assay coefficients of variations (CV) should be less than 5–7%, while inter-assay CVs should be less than 10–15%.

Testosterone can be obtained in serum, saliva and urine. As stated later, we recommend the use of salivary analyses. Nevertheless, some designs make it necessary to use invasive measurements, with testosterone being measured in serum.

Invasive testosterone measurement in serum

The invasive method, where whole blood is collected by venepuncture, is often used in clinical or laboratory settings. Validation studies with intense exercise, for example, are still rare so that it is best to measure saliva and serum simultaneously and compare the results afterwards. In order to quantify the total amount of androgen production, it is also best to measure the total amount of testosterone using invasive measurements in serum. Serum testosterone levels are determined routinely by radioimmunoassays (RIA) or mass spectrometry-based assays (for comparison see Dorgan *et al.*, 2002). The free and the bioavailable testosterone levels which can also be obtained in the serum have been suggested to more reliably represent the bioactive hormone at the tissue level than total testosterone levels (Morley *et al.*, 2002). Direct measurement of free testosterone concentrations (about 2% of the total amount of this steroid), is difficult to do and requires greater assay sensitivity.

Free testosterone can be measured by isotope dilution equilibrium dialysis, the 'gold standard' method (Hackbarth *et al.*, 2011). Equilibrium dialysis is a complex measure of free testosterone in which a blood sample is diluted and passed through a special semi-permeable membrane into a buffer solution. After filtering the sample through this membrane, the amount of testosterone in the buffer solution and the sample is measured and used to calculate the concentration of free testosterone. While this method is considered to be accurate, it is very costly. Immunoassays that detect free testosterone have been proposed as an alternative. However, they have been widely criticized for their lack of accuracy and variability of results with fluctuating SHBG concentrations (Rosner, 2001), suggesting that they do not truly measure free testosterone (Hackbarth *et al.*, 2011).

Another alternative is to calculate free testosterone using equations based on the law of mass action. These equations typically incorporate the results of serum measurements of total testosterone, albumin and SHBG. The calculated results for free testosterone have often been found to vary significantly from isotope dilution equilibrium dialysis (Hackbarth *et al.*, 2011). Thus, we recommend the isotope dilution equilibrium dialysis because it still appears to be the most valid approach for measuring free testosterone in the blood. However, salivary testosterone measured by direct radioimmunoassay offers a simple cheaper alternative to serum free testosterone measurement. All methods – with advantages and recommendations – are described in more detail by Simoni (2004).

Non-invasive testosterone measurement in urine

The determination of testosterone in 24-hour urinary specimens provides the advantage of giving timely and integrated information on levels of secretion (Remer *et al.*, 2005). A mistake in urine collection is one of the most frequent sources of erroneous results, even if the collection procedure has been carefully explained to the participant. An accurate inquiry at the moment of urine delivery to the laboratory can reveal most procedural mistakes (Venturelli *et al.*, 1995). It is widely accepted that the high stability of steroid molecules makes it possible to freeze and store the urine sample at $-20°C$ or less until analysis (Venturelli *et al.*, 1995).

With respect to the analysis of testosterone in human urine, in general immunoassays have been used (Hoffmann *et al.*, 2010). Testosterone in the urine has been estimated by direct immunoassays as well as by RIA in combination with high-performance liquid chromatography (HPLC) purification. Limits of detection (LOD) of 1.5 pg/mL (Bao *et al.*, 2008), 12.2 pg/mL (Al-Dujaili, 2006) or 4.9 pg/mL (Schoneshofer and Weber, 1983) have been reported. Recently, liquid chromatography–tandem mass spectrometry (LC–MS–MS) techniques have been reported, enabling the profiling of testosterone in the urine of adults (Hoffmann *et al.*, 2010). However, by measuring only the urine excretion of testosterone with a lack of plasma or saliva data one cannot determine whether a probable decline of testosterone secretion reflects a reduced production or an increased use.

Non-invasive testosterone measurement in saliva

Testosterone in saliva accurately reflects the unbound, biologically active fraction of testosterone in the general circulation (Granger *et al.*, 1999; Simoni, 2004). A comparison of salivary and serum total or free steroid concentrations shows a significant correlation for almost all salivary steroids (Wood, 2009).

Since free testosterone concentrations represent only a small fraction of the total amounts in serum, salivary assays need to be designed to be ultrasensitive. Available immunoassays with a sensitivity level of 0.8 pg/mL are sufficient to capture nearly 100% of the range of individual differences, even in boys and girls.

For saliva sample collection, it is recommended not to use cotton or polyester swabs (as for example, for cortisol or alpha-amylase) because these tend to increase the measured testosterone levels compared to untreated samples. The impact of oral stimulant interference on testosterone results should also be taken into consideration. Flavoured chewing gums, drinks and food as well as brushing teeth should not be allowed for at least 30 minutes before the data collection. All saliva samples should be frozen first and thawed before assay in order to break down mucopolysaccharides that can interfere with pipetting.

Saliva testosterone levels remain stable for over two years when stored at –80°C. Four weeks in a normal refrigerator (+4°C) can lead to increases of testosterone concentration of about 330%, whereas decreases between 18.2% (–20°C) and 6.5% (–40°C) as well as between 28.1% (–20°C) and 23% (–40°C) can be observed while storing the samples for 6 or 24 months, respectively (Granger *et al.*, 2004). Thus, we recommend analysing testosterone samples promptly without storing them longer than a few days at at least –20°C. If a longer storing time is necessary, samples should be stored at –80°C.

Monitoring testosterone in saliva has several obvious advantages to measurements in serum and urine. By means of saliva collection procedures, researchers are able to conduct repeated sampling over the course of minutes, hours or days. Saliva collection procedures offer more independence and less restrictive circumstances for data collection. Because of its non-invasive character, this method is very convenient and practical even with children. In addition, there is no need for a medical doctor to collect the samples because research assistants and even the participants or their parents can easily collect the saliva samples with the help of minimal instructions. Thus, saliva collection procedures can be recommended, especially for field settings (for a current review see also Gatti and De Palo, 2011).

General note on measurement methods

Before using a commercial kit routinely, in-house revalidation of the candidate assay should be assessed in order to determine its sensitivity, specificity, accuracy and intra-assay precision. Differences between different immunoassays or between immunoassays and the mass spectrometry-based assays often range between –18% and +16% and are even higher for concentrations measured in females or children (Wang *et al.*, 2004; Vesper and Cook Botelho, 2010). To overcome those challenges and to improve the results when comparing measurements using different methods, times and locations, the Steroid Hormone Standardization Project recommends the use of the same kits, procedures and sensitivities for determining testosterone (for more information, see Vesper and Cook Botelho, 2010).

As mentioned above, because testosterone is a small molecule and present in relatively low concentrations, it is not surprising that there is marked inter- and intra-assay bias and variation. Because of the different concentration values of testosterone, this is especially true for the determination in saliva compared to serum and for females and children compared with male samples. Therefore, comparing testosterone levels determined with different assays and/or in different laboratories with different procedures is questionable. Quality control uncovers this problem but has not contributed to its solution (Zitzmann and Nieschlag, 2001). Programmes such as the Steroid Hormone Standardization Project will hopefully improve the comparability in future research.

Interpreting testosterone data

When interpreting testosterone levels it is often overlooked that testosterone levels in body fluids are only one step in the cascade of hormone action from production to biological effect. The primary source of androgens in the male – the Leydig cells – are subject to influence from various substances, such as testosterone itself, oestrogen and glucocorticoids, which are also produced in a diurnal rhythm (see Chapter 3). Thus, when interpreting testosterone data one need to remember that there is a bidirectional link between testosterone levels and an observed behaviour. Thus, changes in testosterone concentration lead to a change in behaviour and vice versa.

All reported variations of testosterone levels and their associations with physical and mental aspects must be viewed critically. The variability in testosterone results and possible differences between measurement methods for free testosterone in saliva and serum (see Granger *et al.*, 2004) can lead to an under- or overestimation of testosterone–behaviour associations in males, and more often in females. This is based on the lower testosterone concentration in females and the resulting higher error rate through the use of equal immunoassay sensitivity for both sexes. Therefore, it is better to analyse only one sex in one study to avoid this problem and to be able to use one special assay regarding the sex of the participants.

Influencing factors of testosterone levels

Sex differences

Androgen receptors are present in many different human system tissues in both males and females. In men, testosterone plays a key role in the development of male reproductive tissues such as the testis and prostate. Furthermore, it is necessary for normal sperm development. In addition, testosterone promotes the secondary sexual characteristics such as increased muscle and bone mass, hair growth as well as deepening of the voice. Like men, women rely on testosterone to maintain libido, bone density and muscle mass as well as erythropoiesis throughout their lives.

In both sexes, the effects of androgens on bone metabolism occur through the same mechanism. Here, testosterone primarily functions by way of aromatization to oestradiol. Aside from maintaining bone mass it accelerates the maturation of cartilage into bone, leading to the closure of the epiphyses and conclusion of growth after puberty (for more detailed information about testosterone and bone metabolism see Zitzmann and Nieschlag, 2004). In the central nervous system, testosterone aromatized to oestradiol serves as the most important feedback signal to the hypothalamus (especially affecting LH secretion, see also Figure 4.1).

Prenatally, at puberty, and throughout life, greatly differing amounts of testosterone account for a variety of biological differences between males and females. Three of these independent periods throughout the life of a human male where testosterone is secreted in increased amounts are noteworthy: (1) during intrauterine life, (2) in the neonatal period, and (3) during puberty. The initial secretory surge in intrauterine life is critical for genital sexual differentiation, whereas the neonatal (and also the intrauterine) surges may play an important role in gender-associated behaviour and structural and functional gender differences in the human brain (e.g. in the hypothalamus, especially the nucleus preopticus, and the limbic system) (Swerdloff *et al.*, 2009). The puberty-caused difference in testosterone concentration between the sexes is shown in Figure 4.3. At approximately the age of 11 or 12 testosterone concentration in boys increases significantly in comparison to that in girls, whose oestrogen levels rise when puberty progresses (see also the following section).

Age differences

At approximately 6 or 8 years of age in both sexes the zona reticularis of the adrenal cortex undergoes maturation (adrenarche) leading to increased

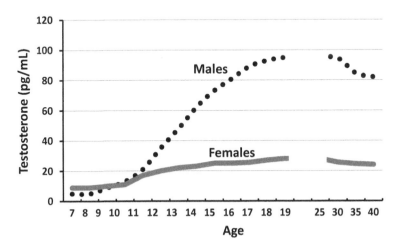

Figure 4.3 Testosterone levels (pg/mL) and age separated for males (dotted line) and females (solid line). Figure 4.3 was created from several data presented in Granger *et al.* (2004).

secretion of androgen precursors (e.g. DHEA). The conversion of these precursors to testosterone and DHT results in the prepubertal growth spurt and the early development of pubic and axillary hair a few years later. The initiation of puberty is determined by an increase in the pulsatile pattern of hypothalamic–GnRH secretion. As puberty progresses, negative feedback sensitivity of the hypothalamus and pituitary to circulating steroids lessens and increasing concentrations of both gonadal steroids and gonadotrophin hormones ensue. Primary and secondary sexual characteristics grow until they reach adult levels.

In early adulthood, serum levels of testosterone reach their peak and begin to decline as early as 30 years of age (see also Figure 4.3). This middle-aged decline in circulating (total and free) testosterone becomes of clinical significance at an older age when circulating levels drop below the threshold for optimal biological functioning. The situation of inadequate androgen secretion and/or sperm production is called hypogonadism. This can be caused by a spectrum of disorders of testicular functions or occur as a consequence of hypothalamic or pituitary failure. It has been shown that with advancing age the proportion of men with testosterone levels in such a suboptimal range increases significantly (e.g. Morley *et al.*, 1997). Low levels can be found in 1% of men aged below 40 years but in 20% of men older than 60 years and in 40% of men above 80 years. These results are confirmed by longitudinal studies (e.g. Morley *et al.*, 1997).

In healthy men, however, the decrease in androgen production is rather a slow process. With age, increased levels of SHBG further decrease the bioavailable testosterone. Reduced levels of growth hormone and insulin-like growth factor 1 (IGF-1), which both inhibit SHBG production in hepatocytes, are responsible for this phenomenon (Vermeulen *et al.*, 1996).

Other influencing factors

Besides age and sex, there are many more factors influencing testosterone levels that also need to be considered when interpreting hormonal data (e.g. Zitzmann and Nieschlag, 2001). In adult men, body mass index (BMI) is negatively correlated with serum testosterone levels (Zitzmann and Nieschlag, 2001): a higher BMI is associated with lower testosterone concentration (e.g. Muller *et al.*, 2003). However, levels of SHBG are also decreased in individuals with high BMI so that bioavailable testosterone remains almost unchanged (Zitzmann and Nieschlag, 2001). Only in extreme obesity (BMI >40 kg/m^2) do testosterone levels decrease to a greater extent than SHBG levels, leading to lower biological functioning. Current tobacco smokers (>5/week) were found to have higher testosterone levels than non-smokers (Muller *et al.*, 2003). Excessive alcohol consumption (>40 g/day) lowers testosterone levels because of its toxic effect on the hypothalamus. Moderate consumption of alcohol (0–40 g/day) does not affect testosterone concentrations (e.g. Muller *et al.*, 2003).

Severe traumatic injuries caused by accidents as well as myocardial or cerebral infarctions, as acutely life-threatening situations cause extreme stress to the individual, leading to high cortisol levels. Because of the close connection between the HPG axis and the HPA axis, pulsatile LH secretion is often (reversibly) diminished in these individuals, leading to clinically lower testosterone concentrations. Other chronic mental (e.g. threatening unemployment) or physical stress situations have been shown to decrease testosterone levels as well. There can also be various reasons for under- or overestimating the effects of exercise on testosterone concentrations.

Social status is described as an influencing factor, too. Schaal and co-workers (1996) found a positive association between high testosterone levels and social dominance but not physical aggression, as assessed by peer ratings. This could suggest that athletes are more likely to have higher testosterone levels because they compete with each other, which might be a sign of social dominance. Similar studies described in the next section discuss the role of winning and losing in sports competitions on testosterone concentrations in men and women.

Physical activity status is also known to influence testosterone concentrations, depending on the duration, intensity and type of physical exercise. In summary, it is important to assess lifestyle factors in testosterone research.

Association with psychological parameters

In the past, testosterone was known to be linked to a few psychological functions such as cognition, aggression, mood and motivation. Yet, findings in the context of sport and athletic competition have not always been consistent (Liening and Josephs, 2010; Helmich et al., 2010). Several of these psychological functions and their biological bases have been proposed as variables that mediate or moderate the interaction between testosterone and behaviour. Liening and Josephs (2010) suggest that two biological mechanisms underlie these influences of psychological variables: first, mechanisms that promote the way testosterone supports approach behaviour by mediation and, second, mechanisms that suppress the way in which testosterone leads to reactive behaviour to social threats.

In men, testosterone effects are promoted when high levels of the peptide hormone vasopressin help to identify socially ambiguous situations (Thompson et al., 2006). In women, in contrast, dominant behaviour is supported when testosterone is metabolized into oestradiol (Trainor et al., 2006; Janowsky, 2006).

An inhibition of the testosterone–behaviour link becomes important when individuals experience threats or need to control impulses. In reaction to a threat, testosterone becomes behaviourally effective when the activation of the HPA axis (cortisol) and serotonergic systems (5-HTTLPR) is low (Viau, 2002; Dickerson and Kemeny, 2004, Helmich et al., 2010). In other words, when exposed to a threat, an individual's behaviour is highly testosterone-driven when cortisol levels are low and the ability to transport (remove) serotonin is high.

Testosterone and cognition

A beneficial relationship between acute physical activity and other measures of academic performance, such as academic achievement in the classroom, might be due to changes in testosterone. In a study with adolescents, Budde and colleagues (Budde *et al.*, 2010b) were able to show that there is a significant rise in testosterone after high but not after moderate exercise intensities. This is of particular interest since testosterone levels (see Hampson, 1995 for review) in young adults have been shown to influence cognitive performance. Studies with healthy young men and women mainly revealed a curvilinear (inverted U-shape) relationship between serum testosterone levels and cognitive functions (Gouchie and Kimura, 1991; Moffat and Hampson, 1996; Muller *et al.*, 2005). High and low levels of testosterone were found to be associated with low spatial ability scores, whereas intermediate levels of testosterone were associated with better spatial performance. Less is known, however, about the link between exercise-related testosterone changes and improved cognitive performance due to acute bouts of exercise. One could assume that the underlying mechanisms of a change in cognitive functions after acute exercise are due to an alteration in testosterone. The inverted U-function between exercise intensity and cognition (Tomporowski, 2003) might be explained by an inverted non-linear function between testosterone and cognitive functioning.

The results of Budde *et al.* (2010b) suggested that 12 minutes of intensive exercise enhanced the testosterone concentration to an extent that it was able to negatively influence working memory performance. This relationship between working memory performance and testosterone level supports the outcomes of the study by Moffat and Hampson (1996), where moderate levels of androgens were associated with better spatial performance. In addition, Wolf and Kirschbaum (2002) reported an increased performance in cognitive tests in men with lower testosterone concentrations. Wolf and colleagues (2000) also reported that the cognitive performance in a verbal fluency task was negatively affected by an acute high dose of testosterone in elderly men. A negative association between testosterone and the working memory task as used by Budde *et al.* (2010b) has not been reported previously. Working memory is mediated, in part, by the prefrontal cortex (Gold *et al.*, 1997). Thus, these results suggest that testosterone might modify the function of this brain region. However, a plausible biological mechanism has not yet been proposed to adequately explain this phenomenon (Beauchet, 2006).

Many of testosterone's behavioural effects occur after it has been converted to its metabolically active derivatives, oestradiol or DHT, by means of the enzymes aromatase and 5α-reductase, respectively (Moffat, 2005). Thus, testosterone may interact not only with androgen receptors (Sternbach, 1998), but also with oestradiol receptors (Moffat, 2005). A possible mechanism for the effects of testosterone on working memory is that testosterone acts via aromatization to oestradiol on the striatal dopamine system with secondary effects on prefrontal functions (Janowsky *et al.*, 2000). At the present time, it is not possible to determine whether testosterone per se is the critical hormone or whether the observed relationships depends on prior conversion to oestradiol and/or DHT.

Testosterone and dominant or aggressive behaviour

In the research on the link between testosterone and externalizing behaviour, dominance refers to a motivation for attaining and maintaining high status within a social hierarchy (Mazur and Booth, 1998). Aggression, in turn, is a specific response to a physical threat (Liening and Josephs, 2010). Meta-analyses repeatedly proposed a small but positive correlation between testosterone and dominant or aggressive behaviour (Book *et al.*, 2001; Archer *et al.*, 2005; Archer, 2006). This correlation is highest among 25- to 35-year-old participants, including athletes and non-athletes. In line with the work of Josephs *et al.* (2003), testosterone's association with dominance is especially pronounced when a participant's self-worth is affected by their performance in a test. This means that people with high testosterone levels have a stronger reaction to situations that challenge their status, which will consequently affect their performance (Archer, 2006).

Other studies have been administered with a focus on physical aggression in competitive sports like martial arts. In judo, for example, higher testosterone levels were correlated with more offensive play in competition. Furthermore, coaches evaluate players high in testosterone more often as looking angry during the fight, being respondent to a challenge or being a violent competitor (Salvador *et al.*, 1987; Archer, 2006). In a subsequent study, Salvador *et al.* (1999) could replicate these findings insofar as those judo players who displayed higher testosterone levels before a competition attacked more often, posed more threat to their opponent and put more effort into fighting to gain advantage during the fight (see also Parmigiani *et al.*, 2006; for women see Bateup *et al.*, 2002). Finally, in studies comparing athletic users and non-users of anabolic steroids, higher levels of aggression were reported for the user group (Choi *et al.*, 1990; Moss *et al.*, 1992; Pope and Katz, 1994).

Testosterone and mood, anxiety or depression

The relationship between internalizing behaviour like depression or anxiety and exercise is often described as being negatively correlated (Daley, 2008). Accordingly, higher testosterone levels are associated with more positive mood and lower levels of anxiety and depression. In hypogonadal and older men, for example, whose testosterone values are more likely to be at the low end of the physiological range, depressive behaviour is found more often. With testosterone substitution, these negative mood stages could be improved (e.g. Barrett-Connor *et al.*, 1999). In adolescent boys, but not girls, Granger and colleagues (2003) found testosterone concentrations lower in participants with more anxiety–depression problems.

Mazur and Lamb (1980) described elevated testosterone levels in participants who had just won a tennis match. However, these increases in testosterone only occurred when participants were proud and happy about their effort and victory. The finding was replicated in a later study by Booth *et al.* (1989), who also found that tennis players showed a rise in testosterone before the match, which was accompanied by positive mood. Salvador *et al.* (2003) showed that testosterone was negatively correlated with negative mood in judo players. In line with this finding, Eubank *et al.* (1997) stated that athletes who perceived their pre-competition anxiety as facilitating showed an increase in testosterone (and lower levels of cortisol) before the competition. In studies in basketball (González-Bono *et al.*, 1999) and judo (Suay *et al.*, 1999), no differences in mood depending on testosterone changes after winning or losing were found.

Testosterone and motivation

Studies on the impact of motivational moderators on the relationship between testosterone and sport performance usually suffer from small sample sizes and inconsistent findings. However, moderating motivational variables can be identified as attribution of success and failure as well as motivation to exert influence on others (the *power motive* – described as the capacity to derive pleasure from having impact on others or to experience the impact of others on oneself as aversive) (Winter, 1973; McClelland, 1975; Liening and Josephs, 2010). In some studies with athletes, differences in testosterone levels could neither be displayed in individuals anticipating a competition (Salvador *et al.*, 2003) nor as a consequence of a competition (Suay *et al.*, 1999). However, in judokas, changes in testosterone levels (from pre- to post-fight) could be associated with their motivation to win (Suay *et al.*, 1999; Parmigiani *et al.*, 2006). The same research group reported that in another judo sample, a certain group of participants who showed increases in anticipatory testosterone also displayed higher motivation to win before the competition (Salvador *et al.*, 2003).

In a chess competition (Mazur *et al.*, 1992) and in wrestling (Elias, 1981) higher levels of testosterone were found in winners and lower levels of testosterone in losers. In a study with female collegiate volleyball and tennis players, Edwards and Kurlander (2010) identified changes in pre- to in-competition testosterone levels. However, these levels did not differ from practice levels of testosterone.

In the light of these inconsistent findings, Schultheiss and Rohde (2002) as well as Wirth *et al.* (2006) suggested that testosterone responses to victory or defeat are moderated by the individual's motivation to exert influence in others (power motive). Only males high in a personalized power motive show raised testosterone levels after victory (McClelland, 1975; Mazur and Booth, 1998). It is assumed that the increase in testosterone levels reinforces the behaviour that leads to the victory (see also Schultheiss *et al.*, 1999, 2005).

In a study in basketball, González-Bono *et al.* (1999) reported that changes in testosterone levels from pre- to post-competition were positively related to an index that explained how many points and playing time the individual contributed to the team performance. In addition, winners who avoided external attribution of their success showed higher testosterone levels.

Other researchers concentrated on whether certain testosterone changes made individuals persevere in subsequent competitions. Mehta and Josephs (2006), for example, found that losers in a puzzle game who showed high levels of testosterone after the competition preferred to compete again over switching to a noncompetitive activity. Carré *et al.* (2010), accordingly, could show that individuals who found it internally rewarding to be reactively aggressive in a computer game also showed higher levels of testosterone. These individuals also preferred to engage in further competition.

Testosterone and sports

There are numerous reports on the effects of physical exercise on testosterone levels and of testosterone on physical performance. While this chapter does not focus on the abuse of androgens to enhance performance and the doping discussion, it should be noted that unfortunately, many of these studies lack control groups, do not have a sufficient number of participants or combine different stressors. In order to systematize the number of studies, we distinguish between endurance and strength training as well as between acute and chronic physical exercise.

Testosterone and endurance sports

The neuroendocrine system, and especially the components that control and regulate the reproductive functions, are extremely sensitive to the stress of physical training. This is true for males and females, although we know much more about males than females. In the following section, we differentiate between physical exercise conducted once (acute bout of exercise) and physical training (chronic bout of exercise) conducted for weeks, months or years, pointing out that the response of the endocrine system differs between these two conditions.

Effects of acute bouts

Acute bouts of exercise cause different effects on testosterone concentration depending on the intensity and duration of the performed activity and the participant's training status. Once a certain threshold, identified as a percentage of maximal aerobic power (Vo_{2max}), is reached, in adults, testosterone levels show significant increases following exercise. In endurance-trained men, 10 minutes of running with 70–80% Vo_{2max} provokes significant increases in total testosterone concentration directly post-exercise (Kenefick *et al.*, 1998). Furthermore, an intense interval exercise protocol produces a 38% rise of total testosterone in trained males (Gray *et al.*, 1993). In this study, after 6 hours of recovery, testosterone concentration decreased significantly under resting levels (16%), pointing to the long-term consequences of endurance exercise.

The rise in hormonal concentration through acute exercise was explained by Arena and Maffulli (2002) through various mechanisms, such as the increasing body core temperature, which interferes with the binding of hormones to plasma proteins accompanied by a consequent increase of the circulating, metabolically active hormonal fraction. Other possible reasons for the acute elevation of plasma testosterone are plasma volume reductions and a reduced hepatic clearance due to a drop in hepatic blood flow or a higher secretion of testosterone through the testes.

In physically healthy active men, a significant increase of free testosterone after

60–90 minutes of different types of endurance exercise of intensities between 65 and 75% Vo_{2max} was shown by Brownlee *et al.* (2005). In young male athletes aged 10–16 years, salivary testosterone also increased by 32% after a 90-minute training session (Di Luigi *et al.*, 2006). In normal high-school students (boys and girls), significant increasing salivary testosterone concentrations have been observed after 12 minutes of exercise at 70–85% of HR_{max} by Budde and colleagues (2010a, 2010b). In exercising women, increasing testosterone concentrations following exercise are also described (see Arena and Maffulli, 2002).

The hormonal response to acute exercise may vary according to the individual's level of training. In trained healthy participants, the reactivity of the HPG axis in response to an acute bout of exercise tends to be more pronounced than in less trained participants, indicating that there is an adaptation to the exposed physical stress situation (Crewther *et al.*, 2011).

As described in Chapter 3, there is a marked relationship between the HPA and HPG axis. The link between the two final hormones – cortisol and testosterone – in response to physical exercise was investigated by Daly *et al.* (2005). They found that directly after an exercise session above 75 minutes until volitional exhaustion endurance-trained males had significant elevated cortisol levels, whereas testosterone levels did not change. During the recovery period, cortisol levels remained high for about an hour. After 90 minutes of recovery, cortisol levels decreased to baseline levels and total and free testosterone levels were significantly lower than at baseline, indicating that there is a negative relationship between the two hormones.

In a study with high-school students, however, this inverse relationship between free testosterone and cortisol after termination of the exercise was not observed after 12 minutes of intense exercise (Budde *et al.*, 2010a, 2010b). The results showed a comparable rise in both steroid hormones. In physically active men, Brownlee and colleagues (2005) found the negative relationship only for total testosterone, but not for free testosterone and cortisol. Interactions between the HPA and HPG axes could be one possible explanation for the long-term effects of exercise on testosterone concentrations (Viau, 2002).

Adaptation to training

Endurance training can have a prolonged effect on androgen levels. Men who participate in endurance exercise events, such as marathons, may perform between 10 and 20 hours of intensive training per week. Controlled trials involving men undergoing such an endurance training and control groups of sedentary men give the impression of generally lowered androgen levels in exercising men (e.g. Hackney *et al.*, 1988). Many male distance runners, through their chronic exposure to endurance training, have developed persistently low basal resting testosterone levels. Several studies have shown a decrease in basal testosterone levels of 20–40% from pre-training levels following one to six months of intensive endurance training (for a review see Hackney, 2008). The majority of these trained men exhibit testosterone concentrations which are at the very low end of the normal range. Only a few of them reach subclinical testosterone concentrations.

Other investigations, conversely, did not report significant changes in basal testosterone concentrations following endurance training periods of between two and twelve months. These differences are explained by the different training status/physical fitness of the participants or they may be linked to the exercise dosage administered within the individual research studies. The underlying mechanisms are not yet totally understood (Hackney, 2008).

Normal feedback regulation would require luteinizing hormone (LH) levels to rise with falling testosterone. Zitzmann and Nieschlag (2001) argued that a suppression in the feedback regulation of the HPG axis could explain why differences in gonadotropin levels (LH and FSH) are rarely seen in exercising versus sedentary men, despite marked differences in testosterone levels (Zitzmann and Nieschlag, 2001). Especially in hypogonadal distance runners, such a lack of increasing basal LH concentration was observed in correspondence with substantially reduced testosterone levels (Hackney, 2008).

Training and competition in physical endurance means exposure to physical stress. Stress can have a negative impact on testosterone secretion through inhibitory actions directly at the Leydig cells of the testes and/or disruption of the HPG regulatory axis. Different reactivity of the HPA axis is seen between so-called high and low responders (Granger *et al.*, 1994). The lowering effect of endurance training on testosterone levels may be seen as part of a general response pattern to repeated physical stress, especially in high cortisol responders (Granger *et al.*, 1994; Crewther *et al.*, 2011).

Decreased basal testosterone levels may have a cardiovascular protective effect and thus positive health consequences for the distance-trained males, as have been shown by Van Eckardstein *et al.* (1997). They found a link between decreased testosterone concentrations and significant increases of high-density lipoprotein (HDL), which is correlated with cardiovascular health.

Testosterone and resistance sports

In men and women, muscle mass and strength are often described as being associated with testosterone levels. This applies to older men and women as well as to adolescents. In the following, we summarize some interesting studies dealing with effects of acute bouts of resistance exercise as well as effects of longitudinal resistance exercise.

Effects of acute bouts

Acute elevations in circulating blood concentrations of anabolic hormones such as testosterone during and immediately following a resistance exercise protocol are very well documented. Resistance exercise has been shown to acutely increase total testosterone concentrations in most studies in young and old men (e.g. Kraemer *et al.*, 1998a; Ahtiainen *et al.*, 2003; Izquierdo *et al.*, 2009; McCaulley *et al.*, 2009). In just a few studies testosterone did not change (Smilios *et al.*, 2003). In contrast, the majority of studies in women found no acute change in testosterone levels (e.g. Häkkinen and Pakarinen, 1995; Kraemer *et al.*, 1998b).

This inability to acutely increase testosterone levels may be a crucial gender difference which originates in adolescence (Kraemer *et al.*, 1998b). The acute response of testosterone to resistance exercise is also influenced by the age, training experience of the individuals and sex, as well as baseline values (for review, see also Kraemer and Ratamess, 2005)

A higher testosterone concentration increases the likelihood of an interaction between the hormone and its specific receptor of the target cells, which initiates, for example, the enhanced muscle protein synthesis. Possible reasons for the acute elevations of plasma testosterone besides plasma volume reductions and a reduced hepatic clearance due to a drop in hepatic blood flow are potential adaptations in testosterone synthesis and/or secretory capacity of the Leydig cells in the testes and also adrenergic stimulation or lactate-stimulated secretion (Ahtiainen *et al.*, 2003).

Adaptation to training

Since a single hypertrophic type of resistance exercise induces increases in serum testosterone concentrations, it is also possible that the magnitude and/or duration of the acute hormone response may change due to prolonged strength training. This could be shown by Kraemer *et al.* (1992) who found a greater acute increase in testosterone response following heavy resistance exercise in well-trained junior weightlifters than that of untrained participants. These results are affirmed by Izquierdo and colleagues (2009), who have shown increased acute testosterone response to resistance exercise after a seven-week training period.

Ahtiainen and colleagues (2003) showed enhanced serum basal testosterone concentrations in male strength athletes after 14 weeks of a strength training programme. Kraemer and collegues (1998b) found the same for untrained men and women after a resistance training period of eight weeks. These response patterns could represent a longer term adaptation to support acute exercise performance. This idea is supported by correlations between testosterone and performance responses to exercise in athletes, but there is a lack of a correlation in non-athletes (see Crewther *et al.*, 2011). However, the concentration in the Ahtiainen *et al.* (2003) study decreased to pre-training levels following an additional training period of seven weeks with a lower training volume. These changes in testosterone concentrations were associated with the total training volume and the development of isometric strength. Individual comparisons also showed that untrained participants who showed greater acute testosterone response after training were also able to gain more muscle cross-sectional area than those with lower response. These findings suggest that serum basal testosterone concentration may be an important factor for strength development.

Summary

Testosterone plays a crucial role in psychoneuroendocrinological research because of its bi-directional link between behaviour and physical performance.

Testosterone concentrations are influenced by age, gender and other influencing factors, such as tobacco smoking, alcohol, diseases, physical activity status and psychological variables. Therefore, lifestyle factors have to be involved in the interpretation of testosterone values. As with other hormones, the use of an adequate sample schedule and appropriate assay sensitivity should be considered. Increased testosterone levels are associated with higher dominant and/or aggressive behaviour, whereas anxiety and/or depression are linked to lower testosterone levels. Cognition and motivation also show correlations with testosterone. Highly trained athletes show altered testosterone levels not only in the basal levels but also in response to an acute stress compared with untrained individuals.

However, there are still many questions related to testosterone. For example, many mechanisms for women and children have been studied insufficiently. Exact results in terms of intensity and duration of physical activity and their effects on HPG axis activity and reactivity are also missing.

References

Ahtiainen, J. P., Pakarinen, A., Alen, M., Kraemer, W. J. and Häkkinen, K. (2003). Muscle hypertrophy, hormonal adaptations and strength development during strength training in strength-trained and untrained men. *European Journal of Applied Physiology*, 89, 555–563.

Al-Dujaili, E. A. (2006). Development and validation of a simple and direct ELISA method for the determination of conjugated (glucuronide) and non-conjugated testosterone excretion in urine. *Clinica Chimica Acta*, 364, 172–179.

Archer, J. (2006). Testosterone and human aggression: an evaluation of the challenge hypothesis. *Neuroscience and Biobehavioral Reviews*, 30, 319–345.

Archer, J., Graham-Kevan, N. and Davies, M. (2005). Testosterone and aggression: a reanalysis of Book, Starzyk, and Quinsey's (2001) study. *Aggression and Violent Behavior*, 10, 241–261.

Arena, B. and Maffulli, N. (2002). Endocrinology changes in exercising women. *Sports Medicine and Arthroscopy Review*, 10, 10–14.

Bao, S., Peng, Y., Sheng, S. and Lin, Q. (2008). Assessment of urinary total testosterone production by a highly sensitive time-resolved fluorescence immunoassay. *Journal of Clinical Laboratory Analysis*, 22, 403–408.

Barrett-Connor, E., von Mühlen, D. G. and Kritz-Silverstein, D. (1999). Bioavailable testosterone and depressed mood in older men: the Rancho Bernardo Study. *Journal of Clinical Endocrinology and Metabolism*, 84, 573–577.

Bateup, H. S., Booth, A., Shirtcliff, E. A. and Granger, D. A. (2002). Testosterone, cortisol, and women's competition. *Evolution and Human Behavior*, 23, 181–192.

Beauchet, O. (2006). Testosterone and cognitive function: current clinical evidence of a relationship. *European Journal of Endocrinology*, 155, 773–781.

Book, A. S., Starzyk, K. B. and Quinsey, V. L. (2001). The relationship between testosterone and aggression: a meta-analysis. *Aggression and Violent Behavior*, 6, 579–599.

Booth, A., Shelley, G., Mazur, A., Tharp, G. and Kittok, R. (1989). Testosterone, and winning and losing in human competition. *Hormones and Behavior*, 23, 556–571.

Brownlee, K. K., Moore, A. W. and Hackney, A. C. (2005). Relationship between circulating cortisol and testosterone: influence of physical exercise. *Journal of Sports Science and Medicine*, 4, 76–83.

Budde, H., Pietrassyk-Kendziorra, S., Bohm, S. and Voelcker-Rehage, C. (2010a). Hormonal responses to physical and cognitive stress in a school setting. *Neuroscience Letters*, 474, 131–134.

Budde, H., Voelcker-Rehage, C., Pietrassyk-Kendziorra, S., Machado, S., Ribeiro, P. and Arafat, A. M. (2010b). Steroid hormones in the saliva of adolescents after different exercise intensities and their influence on working memory in a school setting. *Psychoneuroendocrinology*, 35, 382–391.

Carré, J. M., Gilchrist, J. D., Morrissey, M. D. and McCormick, C. M. (2010). Motivational and situational factors and the relationship between testosterone dynamics and human aggression during competition. *Biological Psychology*, 84, 346–353.

Choi, P. Y. L., Parrott, A. C. and Cowan, D. (1990). High-dose anabolic steroids in strength athletes: Effects upon hostility and aggression. *Human Psychopharmacology: Clinical and Experimental*, 5, 349–356.

Crewther, B. T., Cook, C., Cardinale, M., Weatherby, R. P. and Lowe, T. (2011). Two emerging concepts for elite athletes: The short-term effects of testosterone and cortisol on the neuromuscular system and the dose-response training role of these endogenous hormones. *Sports Medicine*, 41, 103–123.

Daley, A. (2008). Exercise and depression: A review of reviews. *Journal of Clinical Psychology in Medical Settings*, 15, 140–147.

Daly, W., Seegers, C. A., Rubin, D. A., Dobridge, J. D. and Hackney, A. C. (2005). Relationship between stress hormones and testosterone with prolonged endurance exercise. *European Journal of Applied Physiology*, 93, 375–380.

Diamanti-Kandarakis, E. (1999). Current aspects of antiandrogen therapy in women. *Current Pharmaceutical Design*, 5, 707–723.

Di Luigi, L., Baldari, C., Gallotta, M. C., *et al.* (2006). Salivary steroids at rest and after a training load in young male athletes: Relationship with chronological age and pubertal development. *International Journal of Sports Medicine*, 27, 709–717.

Dickerson, S. S. and Kemeny, M. E. (2004). Acute stressors and cortisol responses: a theoretical integration and synthesis of laboratory research. *Psychological Bulletin*, 130, 355–391.

Diver, M. J., Imtiaz, K. E., Ahmad, A. M., Vora, J. P. and Fraser W. D. (2003). Diurnal rhythms of serum total, free and bioavailable testosterone and of SHGB in middle-aged men compared with those in young men. *Clinical Endocrinology*, 58, 710–717.

Dorgan, J. F., Fears, T. R., McMahon, R. P., Aronson Friedman, L., Patterson, B. H. and Greenhut, S. F. (2002). Measurement of steroid sex hormones in serum: a comparison of radioimmunoassay and mass spectrometry. *Steroids*, 67, 151–158.

Edwards, D. A. and Kurlander, L. S. (2010). Women's intercollegiate volleyball and tennis: effects of warm-up, competition, and practice on saliva levels of cortisol and testosterone. *Hormones and Behavior*, 58, 606–613.

Elias, M. (1981). Serum cortisol, testosterone and testosterone-binding globulin responses to competitive fighting in human males. *Aggressive Behavior*, 7, 215–224.

Eubank, M., Collins, D., Lovell, G., Dorling, D. and Talbot, S. (1997). Individual temporal differences in precompetition anxiety and hormonal concentration. *Personality and Individual Differences*, 23, 1031–1039.

Gatti, R. and De Palo, E. F. (2011). An update: salivary hormones and physical exercise. *Scandinavian Journal of Medicine and Science in Sports*, 21, 157–169.

Gold, J. M., Carpenter, C., Randolph, C., Goldberg, T. E. and Weinberger, D. R. (1997). Auditory working memory and Wisconsin Card Sorting Test performance in schizophrenia. *Archives of General Psychiatry*, 54, 159–165.

González-Bono, E., Salvador, A., Serrano, M. A. and Ricarte, J. (1999). Testosterone, cortisol, and mood in a sports team competition. *Hormones and Behavior*, 35, 55–62.

Gouchie, C. and Kimura, D. (1991). The relationship between testosterone levels and cognitive ability patterns. *Psychoneuroendocrinology*, 16, 323–334.

Granger, D. A., Weisz, J. R. and Kauneckis, D. (1994). Neuroendocrine reactivity, internalizing behaviour problems, and control-related cognitions in clinic-referred children and adolescents. *Journal of Abnormal Psychology*, 103, 267–276.

Granger, D. A., Schwartz, E. B., Booth, A. and Arentz, M. (1999). Salivary testosterone determination in studies of child health and development. *Hormones and Behavior*, 35, 18–27.

Granger, D. A., Shirtcliff, E. A., Zahn-Waxler, C., Usher, B., Klimes-Dougan, B. and Hastings, P. (2003). Salivary testosterone diurnal variation and psychopathology in adolescent males and females: individual differences and developmental effects. *Development and Psychopathology*, 15, 431–449.

Granger, D. A., Shirtcliff, E. A., Booth, A., Kivlighan, K. T. and Schwartz, E. B. (2004). The 'trouble' with salivary testosterone. *Psychoneuroendocrinology*, 29, 1229–1240.

Gray, A. B., Telford, R. D. and Weidemann, M. J. (1993). Endocrine response to intense interval exercise. *European Journal of Applied Physiology and Occupational Physiology*, 66, 366–371.

Hackbarth, J. S., Hoyne, J. B., Grebe, S. K. and Singh, R. J. (2011). Accuracy of calculated free testosterone differs between equations and depends on gender and SHBG concentration. *Steroids*, 76, 48–55.

Hackney, A. C. (2008). Effects of endurance exercise on the reproductive system of men: the 'exercise-hypogonadal male condition.' *Journal of Endocrinological Investigation*, 31(10), 932–938.

Hackney, A. C., Sinning, W. E. and Bruot, B. C. (1988). Reproductive hormonal profiles of endurance-trained and untrained males. *Medicine and Science in Sports and Exercise*, 20, 60–65.

Häkkinen, K. and Pakarinen, A. (1995). Acute hormonal response to heavy resistance exercise in men and women at different ages. *International Journal of Sports Medicine*, 16, 507–513.

Hampson, E. (1995). Spatial cognition in humans: possible modulation by androgens and estrogens. *Journal of Psychiatry and Neuroscience*, 20, 397–404.

Helmich, I., Latini, A. S., Sigwalt, A., *et al.* (2010). Neurobiological alterations induced by exercise and their impact on depressive disorders. *Clinical Practice and Epidemiology in Mental Health*, 6, 115–125.

Hoffmann, P., Hartmann, M. F., Remer, T., Zimmer, K.-P. and Wudy, S. A. (2010). Profiling oestrogens and testosterone in human urine by stable isotope dilution/benchtop gas chromatography-mass spectrometry. *Steroids*, 75, 1067–1074.

Izquierdo, M., Ibañez, J., Calbet, J. A. L., *et al.* (2009). Cytokine and hormone response to resistance training. *European Journal of Applied Physiology*, 107, 397–409.

Janowsky, J. S. (2006). Thinking with your gonads: testosterone and cognition. *Trends in Cognitive Sciences*, 10, 77–82.

Janowsky, J. S., Chavez, B. and Orwoll, E., (2000). Sex steroids modify working memory. *Journal of Cognitive Neuroscience*, 12, 407–414.

Jensen, J., Oftebro, H., Breigan, B., *et al.* (1991). Comparison of changes in testosterone concentrations after strength and endurance exercise in well trained men. *European Journal of Applied Physiology and Occupational Physiology*, 63, 467–471.

Josephs, R. A., Neman, M. L., Brown, R. P. and Beer, J. M. (2003). Status, testosterone, and human intellectual performance: stereotype threat as status concern. *Psychological Science*, 14, 158–163.

Kenefick, R. W, Maresh, C. M., Armstrong, L. E., *et al.* (1998). Plasma testosterone and cortisol responses to training-intensity exercise in mild and hot environments. *International Journal of Sports Medicine*, 19, 177–181.

Kraemer, W. J. and Ratamess, N. A. (2005). Hormonal response and adaptations to resistance exercise and training. *Sports Medicine*, 35, 339–361.

Kraemer, W. J., Fry, A. C., Warren, B. J., *et al.* (1992). Acute hormonal responses in elite junior weightlifters. *International Journal of Sports Medicine*, 13, 103–109.

Kraemer, W. J., Häkkinen, K., Newton, R. U., *et al.* (1998a). Acute hormonal response to heavy resistance exercise in younger and older men. *European Journal of Applied Physiology*, 77, 206–211.

Kraemer, W. J., Staron, R. S., Hagermann, F. C., *et al.* (1998b). The effect of short-term resistance training on endocrine function in men and women. *European Journal of Applied Physiology*, 78, 69–76.

Lang, F. and Verrey, F. (2007). Hormone. In R. F. Schmidt and F. Lang (eds), *Physiologie des Menschen*, Volume 30 (pp. 474–502), Heidelberg: Springer Medizin Verlag.

Liening, S. H. and Josephs, R. A. (2010). It is not just about testosterone: physiological mediators and moderators of testosterone's behavioral effects. *Social and Personality Psychology Compass*, 11, 982–994.

Mazur, A. and Booth, A. (1998). Testosterone and dominance in men. *Behavioral and Brain Sciences*, 21, 353–397.

Mazur, A. and Lamb, T. A. (1980). Testosterone, status, and mood in human males. *Hormones and Behavior*, 14, 236–246.

Mazur, A., Booth, A. and Dabbs, J. M. (1992). Testosterone and chess competition. *Social Psychology Quarterly*, 55, 70–77.

McCaulley, G. O., McBride, J. M., Cormie, P., *et al.* (2009). Acute hormonal and neuromuscular response to hypertrophy, strength and power type resistance exercise. *European Journal of Applied Physiology*, 105, 695–704.

McClelland, D. C. (1975). *Power: the inner experience*. Oxford: Irvington.

Mehta, P. H. and Josephs, R. A. (2006). Testosterone change after losing predicts the decision to compete again. *Hormones and Behavior*, 50, 684–692.

Moffat, S. D. (2005). Effects of testosterone on cognitive and brain aging in elderly men. *Annals of the New York Academy of Science*, 1055, 80–92.

Moffat, S. D. and Hampson, E. (1996). A curvilinear relationship between testosterone and spatial cognition in humans: possible influence of hand preference. *Psychoneuroendocrinology*, 21, 323–337.

Morley, J. E., Kaiser, F. E., Perry, H. M. III, *et al.* (1997). Longitudinal changes in testosterone luteinizing hormone and follicle-stimulating hormone in healthy older men. *Metabolism*, 46, 410–413.

Morley, J. E., Patrick, P. and Perry, H. M. III (2002). Evaluation of assays available to measure free testosterone. *Metabolism*, 51, 554–559.

Moss, H. B., Panzak, G. L. and Tarter, R. E. (1992). Personality, mood, and psychiatric symptoms among anabolic steroid users. *American Journal on Addictions*, 1, 315–324.

Muller, M., den Tonkelaar, I., Thijssen, J. H. H., Grobbee, D. E. and van der Schouw, Y. T. (2003). Endogenous sex hormones in men aged 40–80 years. *European Journal of Endocrinology*, 149, 583–589.

Muller, M., Aleman, A., Grobbee, D. E., de Haan, E. H. and van der Schouw, Y. T. (2005).

Endogenous sex hormone levels and cognitive function in aging men: is there an optimal level? *Neurology*, 64, 866–871.

Papacosta, E. and Nassis, G. P. (2011). Saliva as a tool for monitoring steroid, peptide and immune markers in sport and exercise science. *Journal of Science and Medicine in Sport*, 14, 424–434.

Parmigiani, S., Bartolomucci, A., Palanza, P., *et al.* (2006). In Judo, Randori (free fight) and Kata (highly ritualized fight) differentially change plasma cortisol, testosterone, and interleukin levels in male participants. *Aggressive Behavior*, 32, 481–489.

Pope, H. G. and Katz, D. L. (1994). Psychiatric and medical effects of anabolic-androgenic steroid use: A controlled study of 160 athletes. *Archives of General Psychiatry*, 51, 375–382.

Remer, T., Boye, K. R., Hartmann, M. F. and Wudy, S. A. (2005). Urinary markers of adrenarche: reference values in healthy subjects, aged 3–18 years. *Journal of Clinical Endocrinology and Metabolism*, 90, 2015–2021.

Rosner, W. (2001). An extraordinarily inaccurate assay for free testosterone is still with us. *Journal of Clinical Endocrinology and Metabolism*, 86, 2903.

Salvador, A., Simón, V., Suay, F. and Llorens, L. (1987). Testosterone and cortisol responses to competitive fighting in human males: a pilot study. *Aggressive Behavior*, 13, 9–13.

Salvador, A., Suay, F., Martinez-Sanchis, S., Simon, V. M. and Brain, P. F. (1999). Correlating testosterone and fighting in male participants in judo contests. *Physiology and Behavior*, 68, 205–209.

Salvador, A., Suay, F., González-Bono, E. and Serrano, M. A. (2003). Anticipatory cortisol, testosterone and psychological responses to judo competition in young men. *Psychoneuroendocrinology*, 28, 364–375.

Schaal, B., Tremblay, R. E., Soussignan, R. and Susman, E. J. (1996). Male testosterone linked to high social dominance but low physical aggression in early adolescence. *Journal of the American Academy of Child and Adolescent Psychiatry*, 35, 1322–1330.

Schoneshofer, M. and Weber, B. (1983). Specific estimation of fifteen unconjugated, non-metabolized steroid hormones in human urine. *Journal of Steroid Biochemistry and Molecular Biology*, 18, 65–73.

Schultheiss, O. C. and Rohde, W. (2002). Implicit power motivation predicts men's testosterone changes and implicit learning in a contest situation. *Hormones and Behavior*, 41, 195–202.

Schultheiss, O. C., Campbell, K. L. and McClelland, D. C. (1999). Implicit power motivation moderates men's testosterone responses to imagined and real dominance success. *Hormones and Behavior*, 36, 234–241.

Schultheiss, O. C., Wirth, M. M., Torges, C. M., Pang, J. S., Villacorta, M. A. and Welsh, K. M. (2005). Effects of implicit power motivation on men's and women's implicit learning and testosterone changes after social victory or defeat. *Journal of Personality and Social Psychology*, 88, 174–188.

Simoni, M. (2004). Methodology for measuring testosterone, DHT and SHBG in a clinical setting. In E. Nieschlag, H. M. Behre and S. Nieschlag (eds), *Testosterone. Action, Deficiency, Substitution* (pp. 641–664). Cambridge: Cambridge University Press.

Smilios, I., Pilianidis, T., Karamouzis, M. and Tokmakidis, S. P. (2003). Hormonal response after various resistance exercise protocols. *Medicine and Science in Sports and Exercise*, 35, 644–654.

Sternbach, H. (1998). Age-associated testosterone decline in men: clinical issues for psychiatry. *American Journal of Psychiatry*, 155, 1310–1318.

Suay, F., Salvador, A., González-Bono, E., Sanchís, C., Martínez, M., Martínez-Sanchis, S., *et al.* (1999). Effects of competition and its outcome on serum testosterone, cortisol and prolactin. *Psychoneuroendocrinology*, 24, 551–566.

Swerdloff, R. S., Wang, C. and Sinha Hikim, A. P. (2009). Hypothalamic-pituitary-gonadal axis in men. In D. W. Pfaff, A. P. Arnold, A. M. Etgen, S. E. Fahrbach and R. T. Rubin (eds), *Hormones, Brain and Behavior*, Volume 5 (pp. 2357–2393). Riverport, MD: Academic Press/Elsevier.

Thompson, R. R., Goerge, K., Walton, J. C., Orr, S. P. and Benson, J. (2006). Sex-specific influences of vasopressin on human social communication. *Proceedings of the National Academy of Science of the USA*, 103(20), 7889–7894.

Tomporowski, P. D. (2003). Effects of acute bouts of exercise on cognition. *Acta Psychologica (Amst)*, 112, 297–324.

Trainor, B. C., Kyomen, H. H. and Marler, C. A. (2006). Estrogenic encounters: how interactions between aromatase and the environment modulate aggression. *Frontiers in Neuroendocrinology*, 27, 170–179.

Tremblay, M. S., Copeland, J. L. and van Helder, W. (2005). Influence of exercise duration on post-exercise steroid hormone responses in trained males. *European Journal of Applied Physiology*, 94, 505–513.

van Eckardstein, A., Kliesch, S., Nieschlag, E., Chirazi, A., Assmann, G. and Behre, H. (1997). Suppression of endogenous testosterone in young men increases serum levels of high density lipoprotein subclass lipoprotein A-I and lipoprotein(a). *Journal of Clinical Endocrinology and Metabolism*, 82, 3367–3372.

Venturelli, E., Cavalleri, A. and Secreto, G. (1995). Methods for urinary testosterone analysis. *Journal of Chromatography B*, 671, 363–380.

Vermeulen, A., Kaufmann, J. M. and Giagulli, V. A. (1996). Influence of some biological indexes on sex hormone-binding globulin and androgen levels in aging or obese males. *Journal of Clinical Endocrinology and Metabolism*. 81, 1821–1826.

Vesper, H. W. and Cook Botelho, J. (2010). Standardization of testosterone measurements in humans. *Journal of Steroid Biochemistry and Molecular Biology*, 1221, 513–519.

Viau, V. (2002). Functional cross-talk between the hypothalamic-pituitary-gonadal and adrenal axes. *Journal of Neuroendocrinology*, 14, 506–513.

Wang, C., Catlin, D. H., Demers, L. M., Starcevic, B. and Swerdloff, R. S. (2004). Measurement of total serum testosterone in adult men: comparison of current laboratory methods versus liquid chromatography-tandem mass spectrometry. *Journal of Clinical Endocrinology and Metabolism*, 89, 534–543.

Winter, D. G. (1973). *The Power Motive*. New York: Free Press.

Wirth, M. M., Welsh, K. M. and Schultheiss, O. C. (2006). Salivary cortisol changes in humans after winning or losing a dominance contest depend on implicit power motivation. *Hormones and Behavior*, 49, 346–352.

Wolf, O. T. and Kirschbaum, C. (2002). Endogenous estradiol and testosterone levels are associated with cognitive performance in older women and men. *Hormones and Behavior*, 41, 259–266.

Wolf, O. T., Preut, R., Hellhammer, D. H., Kudielka, B. M., Schurmeyer, T. H. and Kirschbaum, C. (2000). Testosterone and cognition in elderly men: a single testosterone injection blocks the practice effect in verbal fluency, but has no effect on spatial or verbal memory. *Biological Psychiatry*, 47, 650–654.

Wood, P. (2009). Salivary steroid assays–research or routine? *Annals of Clinical Biochemistry*, 46, 183–196.

Zitzmann, M. (2011). Exercise, training, and the hypothalamic-pituitary-gonadal axis in men. In E. Ghigo, F. Lanfranco and C. J. Strasburger (eds), *Hormone Use and Abuse by Athletes. Endocrine updates*, Vol. 29, (pp. 25–30). New York: Springer.

Zitzmann, M. and Nieschlag, E. (2001). Testosterone levels in healthy men and the relation to behavioural and physical characteristics: facts and constructs. *European Journal of Endocrinology*, 144, 183–197.

Zitzmann, M. and Nieschlag, E. (2004). Androgens and bone metabolism. In E. Nieschlag, H. M. Behre and S. Nieschlag (eds), *Testosterone. Action, Deficiency, Substitution* (pp. 233–254). Cambridge: Cambridge University Press.

5 Catecholamines

*Martin Schönfelder, Thorsten Schulz
and Jana Strahler*

Catecholamines are sympathomimetic hormones released by the adrenal glands in response to physical activity and emotional stress. They are part of the sympathetic nervous system (SNS) and their most abundant forms are adrenaline, noradrenaline and dopamine. Catecholamines bind to various types of adrenergic receptors consisting of different subgroups. Depending on the receptor type catecholamines induce either stimulating or inhibiting effects on the target tissue or cells where they are expressed.

Increased levels of catecholamines are associated with different kinds of stress factors, which can be induced from psychological stimuli or environmental stressors such as elevated sound levels, intense light, intense exercise, hypoxia injury or low glucose levels in the blood. In addition, catecholamines are able to modulate immune functions as well as the cell counts of circulating blood cells.

The water-soluble catecholamines circulate partly bound to proteins in the bloodstream and have a short half-life of a few minutes. After they have exerted their effects, adrenaline and noradrenaline are broken down via several intermediate products to the end-product of metabolism, vanillylmandelic acid, and excreted in urine. Therefore several body fluids such as saliva, urine and plasma can be used to determine both catecholamines and their metabolites in the human body by using several techniques.

In the context of psychoneuroendocrinology the catecholamines represent an indirect link between metabolic pathways and psychological events. Therefore, a predominant interaction between exercise and sport psychology is obvious.

Physiology, biochemistry and mechanisms

Morphological basics of the autonomic nervous system

The peripheral nervous system is divided into two systems: the *somatic or voluntary nervous system*, controlling skeletal muscles, and the *visceral or autonomic nervous system (ANS)*, controlling involuntary visceral homeostasis. The main functions of the ANS are metabolic, cardiopulmonary, secretory and thermal maintenance in the human organism, including the control of blood pressure, heart rate, respiration rate, digestion and sweating (Thomas, 2011). The neurons of the ANS are located in the spinal cord and brainstem. Autonomic neurons do not connect directly to their destinations. They terminate outside of the central nervous system (CNS) in ganglions, where they are synapsed to postganglionic neurons connecting to respective muscle cells or glands. The central neuron that leads to the ganglion is called the preganglionic neuron.

The ANS is divided into two branches: the *sympathetic* and the *parasympathetic system*. All axons of the preganglionic neurons of the parasympathetic system exit the spinal cord cranially and sacrally. In contrast, the sympathetic axons exits through the thoraco-lumbar region. In both cases, the neurotransmitter between the pre- and postganglionic neurons is acetylcholine (ACh), which binds to a nicotinic ACh receptor. With some exceptions, the sympathetic ganglions are located near the spinal cord and constitute the sympathetic chain. Therefore, the sympathetic wiring occurs far from the point of destination, indicating long postganglionic axons. The wiring of the parasympathetic ganglions, however, is located near the organs to be innervated, resulting in short parasympathetic postganglionic axons.

At the destination organs, the postganglionic axons use different neurotransmitters for signalling. Sympathetic postganglionic synapses discharge the catecholamine noradrenaline (also known as norepinephrine), with the exception of ACh at the sweat glands. The cells of the adrenal medulla, which are innervated by preganglionic sympathetic neurons, are homologous to postganglionic neurons and produce two catecholamines: noradrenaline and adrenaline. The succession of a preganglionic stimulus starts with the adrenal medulla releasing a mixture of adrenaline and noradrenaline in the circulation. Transported by the bloodstream, adrenaline and noradrenaline bind to several subtypes of adrenergic receptor (see Table 5.1 and next section) which are variably expressed by the destination organs (Michelotti et al., 2000). In contrast to the sympathetic system, all parasympathetic axons use ACh for neuronal transmission, activating muscarinic ACh receptors at the postsynaptic membrane.

It was long believed that the sympathetic and parasympathetic systems generally have antagonistic effects on the destination cells or organs, but this is not correct. In fact, the two parts of the ANS collaborate to balance homeostasis. Table 5.1 lists the organs or tissue systems affected by the ANS, illustrating the effects and expressed adrenergic receptors of the different neurotransmitters in the sympathetic and parasympathetic system.

As depicted in Table 5.1, the ANS controls diverse visceral functions, largely below the level of consciousness. The various effects of the ANS on heart rate, digestion, respiration rate, salivation, perspiration, diameter of the pupils, micturition (urination) and sexual arousal result from the receptor interaction of noradrenaline and adrenaline and the ratio of noradrenaline: adrenaline by using different biochemical pathways downstream of the receptor binding.

Table 5.1 Effects of the autonomous nervous system and expression of predominant adrenergic receptor

Organ or system	Target	Parasympathetic	Sympathetic	Adrenergic receptor
Heart	Cardiac output	Decrease	Increase	$beta_1$
	Sinatrial node: heart rate (chronotropic)	Decrease	Increase	$beta_1$
	Ventricular contractility (inotropic)	—	Increase	$beta_1$
	Atrial contractility	Decrease	Increase	$beta_1$
	Atrioventricular (AV) node	AV block	Increase conduction velocity	$beta_1$
Blood vessels	Vascular smooth muscle	Relax	Contract/relax	$alpha_1$/$beta_1$,$alpha_1$
	Renal artery	—	Constrict	$alpha_1$
	Larger coronary arteries	—	Constrict	$alpha_1$+$alpha_2$
	Smaller coronary arteries	—	Dilate	$beta_2$
	Arteries to viscera, skin, brain	—	Constrict	$alpha_1$
	Arteries to erectile tissue	Dilate	Constrict	$alpha_1$
	Arteries to salivary glands	Dilate	Constrict	$alpha_1$
	Hepatic artery	—	Dilate	$beta_2$
	Arteries to skeletal muscle	—	Dilate	$beta_2$
	Veins	—	Constrict/dilate	$alpha_1$+$alpha_2$/$beta_2$
Digestive system	Salivary gland secretion	Stimulates water secretion	Stimulates viscous, increase amylase	$beta_2$
	Parietal cells	Gastric acid secretion	—	—
	GI tract (motility)	Increase	Decrease	$alpha_2$+$beta_1$
	Sphincters of GI tract	Relax	Contract	$alpha_1$
	Glands of GI tract	—	Decreased secretion	—
Metabolic system	Liver	—	Glycogenolysis/-neogenesis	$beta_2$ / $beta_1$,+$beta_3$
	Adipocytes	—	Lipolysis	$beta_2$
	Pancreas: beta cells (insulin)	Increase	Decrease	$alpha_2$
	Pancreas: alpha cells (glucagon)	—	Increase	beta

Organ system	Tissue/Cell		Effect	Receptor
Blood cells	Platelets	—	Aggregate	$alpha_2$
	Mast cells (histamine)	—	Inhibit	$beta_2$
Respiratory tract	Smooth muscles of airway	Contract	Relax/contract	$beta_2$/$alpha_1$
Visual system	Pupil dilator muscle	—	Contract (mydriasis)	$alpha_1$
	Ciliary muscle	Contract (short-range focus)	Relax (long-range focus)	$beta_2$
	Lacrimal glands	Secretion		—
Endocrine system	Adrenal medulla	—	Increased secretion of adrenaline and noradrenaline	Nicotinic ACh receptors
Urinary system	Bladder wall	Contract	Relax	$beta_2$
	Urethral sphincter (internal)	—	Contract	$alpha_1$
	Urethra	Relax	Contract	$alpha_1$
	Kidney (renin secretion)	—	Increase	$beta_1$
	Kidney (sodium retention in tubuli)	—	Increase	$alpha_1$
Reproductive system	Uterus	—	Contract	$alpha_1$
	Vescia seminalis, prostate	—	Contract	$alpha_1$
	Ductus deferens	—	Contract	$alpha_1$
Integumentary system	Sweat gland	—	Secretion	Cholinergic
	M. arrectos pili	—	Contract	$alpha_1$

Table adapted from several authors (Arner, 2005; Garruti et al., 2008; Michelotti et al., 2000; Pereira et al., 2010; Philipson, 2002; Schmidt et al., 2007; Wood, 1999; Zouhal et al., 2008).

Biochemical aspects of catecholamines and adrenergic receptors

Biochemically, adrenaline and noradrenaline are called catecholamines because they could be seen as derivatives of the catechol 1,2-dihydroxybenzol. Catecholamine biosynthesis occurs in adrenergic postganglionic nerve cells as well as in the chromaffin cells of the adrenal medulla (Purves *et al.*, 2007; Kvetnansky *et al.*, 2009). The catecholamines are synthesized from the amino acid tyrosine, originating from the diet or from phenylalanine synthesized in the liver. Ultimately, catecholamine synthesis consists of several enzymatic steps leading to the products dihydroxyphenylamine (L-dopamine), noradrenaline and adrenaline (Joh and Hwang, 1987).

Because of their manifold effects, biosynthesis of the catecholamines needs to be strictly controlled by neuronal and hormonal factors. Both adrenaline and noradrenaline positively feed back to the hypothalamus and the pituitary gland, which increase the release of corticotrophin-releasing hormone (CRH) and adrenocorticotrophic hormone (ACTH), respectively. As a result of this positive feedback mechanism, the levels of adrenaline and noradrenaline continue to rise. But to avoid an overshoot of catecholamine production, the increased adrenaline and noradrenaline reduce the activity of their own metabolic key enzymes by allosteric inhibition.

The secretion of catecholamines is a calcium-induced process triggered by ACh in the preganglionic neurons.

The pleiotropic actions of the catecholamines are realized by the use of different subtypes of adrenergic receptors expressed by the destination cells. The expression of these different adrenergic receptor types in human is depicted in Table 5.1. In addition, the various types of receptors use different signalling pathways within the cells. Different actions of adrenaline and noradrenaline have been recognized for several decades, and there have been many pharmacological studies on the diverse agonists and antagonists of catecholamines, leading to the idea of the existence of different receptor types. Modern molecular techniques support these findings and it has now been found that beneath the two main classes of transmembrane receptors – alpha- and beta- adrenergic receptors – there are several subclasses with distinct tissue-specific isoforms of each class. Table 5.2 lists the receptor subclasses and their specific molecular point of action. Noradrenaline primarily activates alpha-receptors and adrenaline primarily activates beta-receptors. In addition, adrenaline may also act at alpha-receptors (Garcia-Sainz *et al.*, 1999).

Downstream, all of the receptor classes use second messenger pathways, leading to specific intracellular modifications. Here, the different receptors transduce the hormonal signal in a G protein-coupled signal, modulating the activity of specific enzyme cascades of the phospholipase C or the adenylate cyclase pathway.

Catecholamine elimination

The plasma levels of the two catecholamines are quite low: 1 nmol/L (0.2 ng/mL) for noradrenaline and 0.2 nmol/L (0.05 ng/mL) for adrenaline. These low

Table 5.2 Function and molecular mechanisms of adrenergic receptors

Receptor	Signalling pathway	Intracellular signal	Main effect
Alpha$_1$	G protein-transduced activation of phospholipase Cβ	Inositol triphosphate; calcium increase	Glycogenolysis, vasoconstriction (e.g. visceral organs)
Alpha$_2$	Gi protein-transduced inhibition of adenylate cyclase	Decrease of cAMP level	Inhibition of lipolysis; inhibition of insulin secretion
Beta$_1$	Gs protein-transduced induction of adenylate cyclase	Increase of cAMP level	Increase of glycogenolysis and gluconeogenesis in liver; increase of insulin secretion; inotropic (heart)
Beta$_2$	Gs protein-transduced induction of adenylate cyclase	Increase of cAMP level	Increase of lipolysis (adipose tissue), vasodilation in skeleton muscles
Beta$_3$	Gs protein-transduced induction of adenylate cyclase	Increase of cAMP level	Increase of lipolysis and thermogenesis

concentrations are due to presynaptic reuptake and enzymatic elimination, which, in mammals, leads to a short half-life for adrenaline and noradrenaline in the blood plasma. The rapid enzymatic degradation to several inactive metabolites is predominantly driven by the enzymes catechol-O-methyltransferase (COMT) and monoaminoxidase (MAO), leading to the formation of 3,4-dihydroxyman-delate, 3-methoxy-4-hydroxyphenylglycolaldehyde (MHPG or MOPEG) and finally to vanillylmandelic acid (VMA) (Kvetnansky *et al.*, 2009). In the periphery, VMA is the major metabolite of catecholamines, and is excreted unconjugated in the urine. The minor metabolite of adrenaline (although the major one in the central nervous system) is MHPG, which is partly conjugated to sulfate or glucuronide derivatives and excreted in the urine (Eisenhofer *et al.*, 2004; Oeltmann *et al.*, 2004). In sum, both catecholamines and their metabolites can be used in scientific research as potential markers for the stress response in biological fluids and tissues.

Determination and assessment

Measurements of catecholamines and their metabolites (e.g. metanephrines, MHPG) can be made in biological fluids and tissues, providing an important analytical parameter in clinical and laboratory research. Catecholamines and most metabolites can be determined using blood (usually plasma) as well as urine, although VMA can be measured only in 24-hour urine samples.

Various techniques exist to determine the specific analytes. If time and facilities allow, they can be quantified with chromatographic techniques, such as high-performance liquid chromatography (HPLC), gas chromatography (GC), and GC-mass spectrometry (MS). Although these allow measurement with good precision and accuracy (Rosano *et al.*, 1991), the necessary know-how and the time-consuming nature of these analytical procedures has led to the validation of simpler techniques, such as enzyme-linked immunoassay or radioimmunoassay (Wolthers *et al.*, 1997). The use of immunoassays may be an alternative to the laborious HPLC, although the methods need to be evaluated in more detail.

Quantification in urine

While urinary catecholamine measurements are considered suitable for observing changes in sympathoadrenergic tone, rapid changes due to acute exercise or emotional stress may be missed. Furthermore, urinary concentrations of adrenaline and noradrenaline have to be related to total urine volume or to a reference substance such as creatinine. Creatinine is a spontaneously formed cyclic derivative of creatine. It is usually produced at a fairly constant rate by the body and eliminated by the kidneys. This is known as creatinine clearance. Creatinine can be used as a reliable standard to control for the possible effects of diet on results since it is not affected by dietary intake (Delanghe *et al.*, 1989).

There are also clear advantages of urinary measurements in psychoneuroendocrine research: urine samples are relatively easy to collect, cause no pain or harm, and in field studies they do not influence the individual's normal behaviour or environment.

Quantification in blood plasma

Plasma levels reflect short-term and acute stress responses more easily than do urinary measurements. The invasive sampling of blood is mainly applied in clinical and laboratory settings. In the ideal case, subjects have to lie still and relax for 30 minutes before and during blood sampling because short periods of standing will alter plasma catecholamines (Kohrt *et al.*, 1993). Samples need to be cooled during transport and have to be analysed within 2 hours of sampling. This circumstance is challenging in research fields such as health or sport science and requires more convenient, non-invasive methods such as saliva sampling.

Quantification in saliva

Catecholamines are readily detectable in saliva but, unfortunately, acute changes in sympathetic activity are not reflected in saliva samples, as diffusion of blood noradrenaline into saliva takes about an hour (Kennedy *et al.*, 2001). In contrast, strong correlations have been observed between plasma and saliva levels of some catecholamine metabolites, including MHPG and VMA (Drebing *et al.*, 1989). MHPG has been related to some aspects of mental health (Li *et al.*, 2006) and could potentially provide an easily obtainable non-invasive marker of acute responses to stress (Okamura *et al.*, 2010).

Confounding factors

When interpreting both integrated measurements for extended periods of time (urine) and acutely altered levels of catecholamines (blood, saliva), one has to be aware that concentrations are subject to various influencing factors as discussed in this chapter. Catecholamines have a pronounced diurnal rhythm, with highest values in the middle of the day and steadily decreasing values with lowest values during night sleep. Other important non-psychological factors influencing both the release and the analysis of catecholamines are caffeine, alcohol, nicotine and drugs (e.g. Jones, 2008), and to a lesser extent food intake, gender, ageing, body weight and phase of menstrual cycle. Finally, a distinct catecholamine response has been found related to physiological states, such as hypoglycaemia (Nordin, 2010), hypoxia (Wheatley *et al.*, 2011) and acidaemia (Ingemarsson, 2003). For scientific research as well as medical diagnostics it is important to note that there is considerable inter-individual variation in baseline levels, while within-subject levels are relatively stable over time (Forsman and Lundberg, 1982). The physiological responses are also associated with the psychosocial working environment (Hansen *et al.*, 2009).

Psychological correlates of catecholamine output

There is strong evidence that psychological factors are heavily correlated with circulating catecholamines. Anxiety, mental stress and pain, including anticipation of pain, all increase circulating catecholamine levels (Hjemdahl *et al.*, 1986; Bremner *et al.*, 1996; Pacak and Palkovits, 2001; Harden *et al.*, 2004). In studies on catecholamine responses it has been found that final exams in college students, occupational job strain, playing a video game or sleep deprivation all revealed increased catecholamine levels (Dimsdale and Moss, 1980; van Doornen and van Blokland, 1989; Stock *et al.*, 1993; Irwin *et al.*, 1999) and there was a positive correlation between subjective arousal and catecholamine secretion during exams (Sherman *et al.*, 2009). In particular, naturalistic stressors that are characterized by uncertainty (Frankenhaeuser, 1971) and that elicit anxiety increase catecholamine excretion (James *et al.*, 1989).

There is evidence that both sensory overstimulation but also deprivation elevates catecholamine output (Frankenhaeuser, 1975). The latter finding has been discussed in the light of isolation or confinement associated with sensory deprivation (Goldberger, 1993). Furthermore, catecholamines are related to the nature of the stimulus and to individual characteristics such as personality type, motivation, experience and attitude (Sokolov *et al.*, 1983). Several situational characteristics determine catecholamine release, including novelty (Mason, 1968) and social and cultural factors such as threat (Lazarus and Folkman, 1984) and perceived control (Dohrenwend and Dohrenwend, 1970).

With respect to personality factors, the literature on extraversion-related differences is controversial, with some authors reporting positive correlations between extraversion scores and MHPG, measured in cerebrospinal fluid (Roy *et al.*, 1989), whereas others report equivalent basal and stress-induced values (Netter *et al.*, 1994). Much of the personality research focuses on type A behaviour, characterized by irritability, hurried behaviour, work achievement and competitiveness. Higher type A behaviour was shown to be related to lower daytime urine concentrations of noradrenaline (Lambert *et al.*, 1987) and adrenaline (van Doornen and van Blokland, 1989). Higher competitiveness also predicted lower night levels of noradrenaline in men and lower daytime levels in women (Lambert *et al.*, 1987).

Using the Karolinska Scale of Personality, Flaa *et al.* showed that catecholamines at rest and during stress are clearly related to multiple personality traits such as detachment (a need to remain distant and a fear of closeness), irritability or verbal aggression (Flaa *et al.*, 2007). Furthermore, plasma adrenaline was positively correlated with psychometric measures of depression, high somatic focus, avoidant coping style and emotional sensitivity/suspiciousness ('paranoia/hostility'). In contrast, no significant correlations were demonstrated with noradrenaline levels (Harden *et al.*, 2004).

Catecholamine responses to exercise

Catecholamines and energy demand

Metabolism represents the sum of chemical reactions in a living organism. Metabolic reactions take place in an organism, no matter what stage predominates, rest or exercise and the metabolic pathways are controlled on the enzymatic level or by different kinds of hormones. Factors affecting metabolism include exercise as well as growth, food consumption, starvation, stress or disease (Mougios, 2006). Without doubt, exercise is one of the most potent effectors of metabolism, representing the following modulations:

- Exercise metabolism follows increased energy needs.
- Exercise affects metabolism not only in contracting muscles but also in other organs (e.g. liver and adipose tissue).
- In most cases of exercise the breakdown of energy sources is increased (carbohydrates, lipids and in some degree amino acids).
- Exercise affects metabolism in an acute, postexercise and chronic manner possibly inducing different profiles.

Several hormones work to facilitate glucose and free fatty acid (FFA) availability, facilitating energy demands, especially in the acting muscles to maintain adenosine triphosphate (ATP) levels. Four hormones are responsible for the increase of plasma glucose level: glucagon, cortisol and the two catecholamines adrenaline and noradrenaline. At rest, glucose release from the liver is initiated by glucagon, leading to increased glycogenolysis as well as the promotion of gluconeogenesis out of glucogenic amino acids (Brosnan, 2003). The maintenance of glucose levels during exercise is facilitated by an increase of glucagon supported by an elevation of catecholamines from the adrenal medulla, further enhancing glycogenolysis. The extent of glucose liberation depends on both the exercise intensity and the duration. Therefore, the catecholamine release increases with elevation of the intensity (Mougios, 2006).

The molecular basis of glucose regulation by catecholamines combines two principles. First, in the acting muscle the adrenergic effect is driven by the binding of adrenaline to beta-adrenergic receptors (see also Table 5.2), leading to activation of the glycogen phosphorylase and in parallel to an inhibition of glycogen synthase (Mougios, 2006). Second, adrenaline binds to another type of receptor in the liver, the alpha$_1$-adrenergic receptor (see also Table 5.2), inducing a different cascade compared to the muscle. This activation finally induces the activity of the enzyme glycogen phosphorylase. The antagonist of glucagon and adrenaline in the case of plasma and muscle glucose homeostasis is insulin; glucagon and adrenaline increase glucose level, whereas insulin signals a decrease. Conversely, high glucose levels negatively feed back on production of adrenaline and glucagon and positively on insulin secretion.

As mentioned above, exercise not only speeds up glycogenolysis but also the process of FFA mobilization, a process called *lipolysis*. Lipolysis in the adipocytes is triggered by adrenaline from the adrenals, noradrenaline from the endings of sympathetic nerves and insulin from the pancreas. Comparable to glycolysis, in the case of lipolysis adrenaline and noradrenaline serve as agonists and insulin as antagonist, which is realized by interaction of the different intracellular signalling cascades (Mougios, 2006).

Beyond energy supply, catecholamines also support oxygen delivery by modulating the affected oxygen related transport pathways. Thus, catecholamines positively affect:

- oxygen transport in respiratory organs by relaxing smooth muscles of bronchioles;
- increased cardiac output;
- vasodilatation in the working muscle; and
- redistribution of blood volume from the intestine organs in favour of working muscles.

In sum, we see that the catecholamines adrenaline and noradrenaline together with glucagon, cortisol and insulin play the major role in hormonal regulation of energy demand. The orchestration of up- and down-regulation of several second messenger principles reflects the fine tuning of metabolic reactions at rest as well as during exercise.

Catecholamines and exercise, training and gender

As we have seen, the stress hormones adrenaline and noradrenaline are responsible for many metabolic adaptions. Therefore, a lot of studies have focused on these amines and their function, especially adaptive processes in exercise, training and gender which represent the main focus in the present subsection. These adaptive processes have been intensively studied and reviewed by Zouhal and colleagues (Zouhal et al., 2008). In addition, catecholamine response to non-exercise-related stressors such as psychosocial stressors has also been noted.

Exercise and catecholamine response

Just as the characteristics of physical exercise are varied, so are the sympathoadrenal responses. The catecholamine response and therefore also the quantification of adrenaline and noradrenaline are dependent on a variety of factors, such as body posture, type of exercise, duration, intensity and catecholamine clearance.

In the context of body posture, most authors agree that in untrained subjects catecholamine levels at rest (sitting or lying) are lower than those in standing posture (Kohrt *et al.*, 1993). For adrenaline, an increase of almost 40% on resting levels could by measured in an upright posture. In addition, several authors found higher noradrenaline levels at a given exercise intensity in an upright posture compared to in a lying position (Christensen and Brandsborg, 1973).

Some authors have postulated an adaptive process in trained subjects, indicating no significant changes in catecholamine concentration in dependency of the body posture (Bloom *et al.*, 1976; McCrimmon *et al.*, 1976).

Different physiological responses concerning heart rate and ventilation have been found when dynamic exercise is carried out at a given oxygen uptake with either the upper or lower body (Blomqvist *et al.*, 1981). Potentially, the effect is based on the mass of the active muscle mass. If the exercise is performed with the upper body (arms) the active muscle mass is lower than if done with the legs. Therefore, the effective workload in smaller muscles is higher than in larger muscles. This circumstance could lead to a higher sympathoadrenal activity, leading to an increase in circulating catecholamines which has been shown by several authors (Kjaer *et al.*, 1987).

Classical endurance disciplines such as swimming, cycling and running represent dynamic or cyclic movement. In addition, there are also some kinds of sports which are characterized by static exercise or isometric muscle contractions. High intense static exercise is accompanied by a more or less permanent compression of the intramuscular vessels. Consequently, the blood in the acting muscle is reduced, representing an additional hypoxic stressor. This makes a direct comparison of static and dynamic exercise difficult. Nevertheless, it is known that plasma catecholamine concentrations increase markedly in men during dynamic (Galbo *et al.*, 1975) and static exercises (Vecht *et al.*, 1978). In the case of dynamic exercise the intensity of the exercise has to exceed a critical level of about 30 beats/minute or 30% of the relative Vo_{2max} (Christensen and Brandsborg, 1973).

The critical level of intensity could differ between noradrenaline and adrenaline. Several authors have mentioned that noradrenaline elevation possibly occurs at lower intensity than necessary for a significant increase of adrenaline. In the case of isometric exercise, several studies have produced inconsistent results. Most of the authors postulate an increase of both catecholamines, whereas others describe a predominant increase of adrenaline. In contrast to these findings, some authors did not find any alteration of catecholamine levels in response to static exercise, as reviewed by Zouhal and colleagues (Zouhal *et al.*, 2008).

Further modulators of catecholamines are the duration and intensity of the exercise. The time-dependent effect of exercise on catecholamine levels mirrors a continuous increase of adrenaline and noradrenaline with the duration of the exercise (Friedmann and Kindermann, 1989). Horton and co-workers describe this increase in catecholamines for low intensity exercise as well, although in this case noradrenaline elevated more quickly than adrenaline (Horton *et al.*, 1998).

Almost all studies dealing with the influence of exercise intensity have found a catecholamine elevation with increasing intensities. But in direct comparison of the studies the range of postulated increases is quite high. This high variation of the results is possibly because of several factors in the study designs: the physical fitness of the participants, the duration of the exercise and also the difference in activated muscle mass. In addition, the time point of blood sampling could also be a critical factor for interpreting absolute catecholamine concentrations.

Gender aspects of catecholamines

In the context of catecholamine response to exercise, Zouhal and colleagues have intensively reviewed the specific gender aspects (Zouhal *et al.*, 2008). They conclude narratively that most of the analysed studies have shown a higher post-exercise adrenaline concentration in endurance-trained subjects in response to intense exercise. The development of a so-called 'sports adrenal medulla' corresponds to the increased secretory capacity of adrenaline liberation in trained versus untrained persons (Kjaer, 1998). In contrast to men, studies on women have shown no evidence that aerobic exercise training affects catecholamine response. It has to be noted, however, that additional studies are necessary to clear this statement. In men, an anaerobic training regime increases the secretory capacity for adrenaline. Furthermore, recent studies suggest that anaerobic training possibly increases this capacity more than aerobic training. Additional studies are indicated in women.

Although further studies on sex differences in exercise response are needed, it is apparent that gender differences in catecholamine response are probably located much earlier in life. Ingemarsson (2003) studied the gender aspects of preterm births and found that the death rate is higher for male than for female fetuses. In 1993, the overall 1-year mortality rate over all gestational weeks in Sweden was 5.4% for boys and 4.1% for girls. The release of catecholamines during labour is an important defence mechanism for a hypoxic fetus. The finding that preterm females show significantly higher catecholamine levels than males possibly indicates that females may be better prepared for hypoxic events than their male counterparts.

Age effects

Beyond the possible gender differences, the ageing of the sympathoadrenal system is much more evident. Systematic experimental approaches indicate that the activity of the tonic whole-body SNS increases with age (Seals and Esler, 2000). In contrast, it is initially surprising that the secretion of adrenaline from the adrenal medulla is markedly reduced with age. But this circumstance is reversed by the reduction of the catecholamine clearance rate. Thus, plasma levels of adrenaline are almost unchanged. Seals and Esler postulated that the mechanisms underlying the age-associated increases in SNS activity are based on an increased subcortical central nervous system sympathetic drive.

With ageing, there are natural changes in the cardiovascular system. These should be differentiated from the effects of pathology, such as coronary artery disease, which occur with increasing frequency as age increases (Cheitlin, 2003). In addition, there is decreased responsiveness to beta-adrenergic receptor stimulation, a decreased reactivity to baroreceptors and chemoreceptors, and an increase in circulating catecholamines. These changes set the stage for isolated systolic hypertension, diastolic dysfunction and heart failure, atrioventricular conduction defects and aortic valve calcification – all diseases seen in the elderly.

Furthermore, because of the interaction of the sympathoadrenal system with the fat stores, leptin secretion and adrenocortical androgen production, Weise and colleagues postulate a possible role in sexual maturation (Weise *et al.*, 2002). They have shown that adrenaline and its metabolite metanephrine decreased significantly with advancing puberty and levels were higher in boys than in girls. In addition, adrenaline and metanephrine are correlated inversely with dehydroepiandrosterone sulfate, oestradiol, testosterone, leptin and insulin.

Long-term adaptation to chronic physiological stress

As already discussed, exercise represents a physical stress that threatens homeostasis and triggers responses of the ANS, including the elevation of catecholamine concentration in plasma (Friedmann and Kindermann, 1989). During long-term endurance training, there seems to develop an enhanced adrenaline responsiveness from the adrenal medulla illustrated in an hypoxia-induced higher adrenaline response, but only in trained athletes (Kjaer *et al.*, 1988). In addition, a second bout of exercise on the same day results in a more pronounced catecholamine response (Ronsen *et al.*, 2001). In contrast, plasma catecholamines were found to rise significantly less in athletically trained compared to untrained subjects (Bloom *et al.*, 1976). Moreover, this effect seems to be specific for noradrenaline while no significant training-induced differences were found for adrenaline (Chwalbinska-Moneta *et al.*, 2005). These findings questions adaptive processes of the catecholamine stress response to exercise as a result of physical training.

There is even evidence that the catecholamine response to acute physical stress rises for adrenaline at exercise workloads over 60% of Vo_{2max} (Frankenhaeuser, 1991; Webb *et al.*, 2008) and for noradrenaline a curvilinear increase to enhanced workloads was observed, although the chronic adaptations remain unclear. Guezennec *et al.* (1986) suggested that in weightlifters studied for four months, training reduces the catecholamine response to resistance exercise.

In our own study, we made a weekly measurement of basal catecholamine levels in cyclists over a period of six months. On average, they had a training volume of over 8000 km on the bicycle. Over the period, the catecholamine concentration remained unchanged, while cortisol levels were chronically elevated (Schulz, 2002).

Sport as a psychological stressor

In addition to physical strain during exercise, the mental stress of, for example, competition and associated emotions has an effect on the secretion of catecholamines. These psychological effects of physical activity led to the suggestion that noradrenergic systems subserve antidepressant effects. Harte and Eifert (1995) showed that environmental setting, subjects' attentional focus and cognitive appraisal all have decisive effects on emotional experiences associated with physical activity. For instance, while indoor running induced a less positive mood, outdoor running resulted in subjects feeling less anxious, less depressed, less hostile, less fatigued and more invigorated, with lower noradrenaline levels but no differences in adrenaline secretion.

Moreover, there is evidence that adrenaline and noradrenaline might be selectively related to different emotional states elicited during physical and psychological stress. While passive, tense and anxious reactions are characterized by heightened adrenaline secretion, responses associated with active aggression predominantly raise noradrenaline levels (Funkenstein, 1956). Assessing the effects of real compared to simulated competition, Guezennec *et al.* (1992) found higher adrenaline (5.3-fold) and noradrenaline (3.7-fold) values before a real pistol-shooting competition. However, only noradrenaline was increased during the shooting. This increase might be a response to mental stress, upright posture and isometric muscle activity, which have been shown to have differential effects on adrenaline and noradrenaline (Taggart and Carruthers, 1971; Galbo, 1983; Jörgensen *et al.*, 1985).

In studies of habituation to stress, it was suggested that catecholamine levels are directly proportional to subjective emotional responses (Salmon, 1992) and that there is a decrease of responses with repetition (Frankenhaeuser *et al.*, 1962). Adrenaline levels may be increased in response to situations characterized by novelty and uncertainty (e.g. real competition), while conditions that are familiar and stereotyped mainly activate noradrenaline (Frankenhaeuser, 1971).

Sport, fitness and stress reactivity

The effect of fitness level on stress responses to psychological stimuli and the effect of acute physical activity on subsequent responses to mental stress is another issue of interest. Two adaptive processes are discussed: habituation reflected in attenuated responses and sensitization reflected in enhanced responses. The effects of acute exercise on psychosocial stress responses have been well studied (for reviews see Taylor, 2000; Boutcher and Hamer, 2006) and hint towards a reduced stress reactivity in >20 minute and >60% Vo_{2max} exercise regimes. Examining the effects of habitual training and aerobic fitness on stress reactivity to cognitive and psychosocial stress has also been extensively studied. As already mentioned, there seems to be a dissociation between adrenaline and noradrenaline, with noradrenaline but not adrenaline reactivity being attenuated in high-fit subjects compared to low-fit subjects, accompanied by a sustained cognitive performance during a vigilance task (Sothmann *et al.*, 1987) or mild psychological stress (e.g. Stroop Conflicting Color Word Task, Péronnet *et al.*, 1989). However, the use of aerobic training for reducing catecholaminergic activity during psychological stress was also questioned (Sothmann *et al.*, 1991, 1992).

Overall, numerous reviews and meta-analyses have been produced, albeit with contradictory findings (Crews and Landers, 1987; Holmes, 1993; Jackson and Dishman, 2006; Sothmann, 2006). Results show that trained individuals have a marginally increased stress response and an improved and faster stress recovery. However, this is primarily true for heart frequency, blood flow and electrodermal activity, while there is no effect of fitness level on catecholamines. Furthermore, there is evidence that subjects in poor health may well benefit from physical activity (Schuler and O'Brien, 1997).

Catecholamines and immune response

Beyond exercise, the greatest stressors for an organism are trauma or illness (Cohen, 2002). Also in this context the stress hormone response mediated by the hypothalamic–pituitary–adrenal (HPA) axis is a part of the normal response to injury. Therefore, the catecholamine elevation is a typical physiological stress response to sepsis, trauma or surgery. For example, Juma *et al.* (1991) noted elevated catecholamine levels within the first 24 hours after orthopaedic surgery. The catecholamine elevation in response to physiological (but also psychological) stressors in turn has effects on the system that keeps people healthy – the immune system. Thus it is clear that the catecholamines play a central role in the interaction and regulation of the communication systems of the body.

The immune system

Beside the two central communication systems of the human body – the nervous and the hormone systems – a third basic information and surveillance system developed during the phylogenesis of humanity in the human organism: the immune system (Ferenčík *et al.*, 2006). For a long time, all three systems were considered to be separate structures (Ader *et al.*, 1995; Besedovsky and Del Rey, 1996; Delves *et al.*, 2011), but it is now known that they share some of the classic basic information molecules for networking as described previously.

Typical messengers in this psycho-neuro-endo-immune networking are the neurotransmitters, cytokines, neuropeptides and different hormones (Ferenčík *et al.*, 2006). More than 100 of those messengers have been described (Delves *et al.*, 2011; Souza-Moreira *et al.*, 2011). In this context, stress hormones and in particular catecholamines play a prominent role. All the messengers of the nervous system, the hormone system and the immune system not only transduce their information via the specific receptor interactions within their particular system, they also act as alternative mediators in the communication process between the three systems (Malarkey and Mills, 2007). Thus both the nervous system and the endocrine system have immunomodulatory effects, whereas the immune system can act as a sensory organ. It is able to recognize specific stimuli that cannot be detected through the central or the peripheral nervous systems. They thus have an increasingly important role in diagnostic, preventive and clinical medicine, in sport science and of course psychology (Ferenčík *et al.*, 2006).

The immune system is a functional unit that consists of different organs, tissues and circulating cells. The lymphatic system represents the organs and tissues: for example the spleen, the tonsils, the thymus, the red bone marrow or the lymph nodes (Berczi *et al.*, 2009). A further special tissue in the sense of physiology is the blood, which carries dissolved immunoglobins (antibodies) and the complement system. Cellular components are the white blood cells. These can be divided into monocytes; eosinophil, basophil and neutrophil granulocytes; lymphocytes and their related plasma cells; as well as the dendritic cells (Ferenčík *et al.*, 2006; Murphy *et al.*, 2009). All these structures work together to maintain the health of the human body and protect it against foreign organisms. As a dynamic regulation system it is persistently exposed to multiple stressors. These stressors affect the homeostasis of the immune system.

Using the CD (cluster of differentiation) nomenclature, all immune cells can be differentiated into further subpopulations. For example all T lymphocytes are identified by expression of the CD3 surface molecule, whereas natural killer cells (NK cells) are determined by the detection of CD16+/56+ molecules (Janeway and Travers, 1995; Roitt *et al.*, 1995).

As described below, the stress hormones adrenaline and noradrenaline are especially immunological relevant (Rabin *et al.*, 1996; Schedlowski *et al.*, 1996).

Catecholamines and immune functions

The influence of adrenaline on circulating white blood cells has been known since the early twentieth century. In 1904 Loeper and Crouzon descibed a so-called 'leucocytosis' induced by adrenaline (Loeper and Crouzon, 1904). During a leucocytosis enhanced counts of white blood cells could be detected in the blood, with increased levels up to 300% and more. The measured leucocytosis was induced by an increase of lymphocytes and neutrophil granulocytes, a so-called lymphocytosis or granulocytosis. Today, an enhanced cardiac output and blood pressure has been described for lymphocytosis, with a significant increase in NK cells and CD8+ cells (Gabriel, 2000). Still, it is clearly demonstrated that the mobilization of the lymphocytes and consequently the appropriate subpopulations are affected by catecholamines (Shepard, 2003). The catecholamines bind to adrenergic receptors expressed on the surface of the lymphocytes, inducing the mobilization of lymphocytes into the circulation (Ahlborg and Ahlborg, 1970; French *et al.*, 1971; Muir *et al.*, 1984; Tonnesen *et al.*, 1987; Brohee *et al.*, 1990; Schedlowski *et al.*, 1996). Especially beta$_2$-adrenergic receptors were expressed in a cell-specific manner correlating to the levels of several lymphocyte subpopulations in the bloodstream (Khan *et al.*, 1986; Maisel *et al.*, 1989; van Tits and Graafsma, 1991; Mond *et al.*, 1995; Rabin *et al.*, 1996).

As previously described, noradrenaline activates primarily alpha- and beta$_1$-adrenergic receptors, whereas only minor effects of noradrenaline on beta$_2$-adrenergic receptors has been reported. In contrast, adrenaline stimulates the beta$_2$-adrenergic receptors to a high extent. The inhibition of adenylate cyclase decreases the intracellular cAMP concentration in lymphocytes (Motulsky and Insel, 1982; Benschop *et al.*, 1996), which finally leads to a short-term modification of the adhesion receptors and consequently to a detachment from the endothelial cells of the blood vessels, the spleen or other lymphatic organs (Benschop *et al.*, 1993, 1994; Lub *et al.*, 1995). In conclusion, stress-induced release of adrenaline results in a beta$_2$-adrenergic receptor-mediated leucocytosis with a fast lymphocytosis. It has been suggested that this could be the result of a short-term support of a physiological evolutionary relic: the fight-or-flight response (Segerstrom and Miller, 2004).

In correspondence with the blood concentrations, catecholamines provoke the flushing of white blood cells into the blood flow and stimulate the activity of the immune cells (Rabin *et al.*, 1996). For example, high levels of adrenaline restrain the proliferation of lymphocytes or an expression of interleukin 2 (IL-2) receptors on lymphocytes induced by mitogens. Also the CD4+ T cells have been found to be lowered by the secretion of IL-2 following high doses of adrenaline (Crary *et al.*, 1983; Khan *et al.*, 1986; Conlon *et al.*, 1988). Both the IL-2 receptor and its ligand play a significant role in the activation of the immune cells, especially the cytotoxic NK cells, lymphokine-activated killer cells (LAK cells) and activated macrophages. IL-2 is a member of the interleukin family which belongs to the class of the cytokines that regulate the proliferation and development of cells.

There are various reports on the effect of high levels of adrenaline on the cytotoxicity of NK cells. Some authors describe an enhanced cytotoxicity of the NK cells against tumour cells, while others refer to a reduced cytotoxicity (Hellstrand *et al.*, 1985; Tonnesen *et al.*, 1987; Kappel *et al.*, 1991; Schedlowski *et al.*, 1993, 1996). Also the evidence for the oxidative burst activity of neutrophil granulocytes is controversial: Berczi (1997) referred to a reduced activity and Burns *et al.* (1997) and Suzuki *et al.* (1999) found an enhanced activity. However, high levels of adrenaline lowered chemotactic behaviour (Davis *et al.*, 1991) and reduced antiviral and tumour cell killing attributes of macrophages (Conlon *et al.*, 1988; Dantzer and Kelley, 1989). In a long-term study over six months, collecting 37 blood samples between 7.30 a.m. and 8.30 a.m., we found a negative correlation of adrenaline and the monocyte phagocytosis (Schulz, 2002).

The administration of noradrenaline has been reported to lead to an increased lysis activity of NK cells in whole blood (Kappel *et al.*, 1998), without affecting the lysis activity of the single NK cell. Higher rates of the lysis through the NK cells in the whole blood could be explained by the elevated cell counts after the catecholamine-induced mobilization.

In summary, in the long term and at high concentrations adrenaline is found to have immune suppressive properties related to the most important immune cells.

Because of their short half-life, the concentration of the catecholamines decreases relatively quickly after specific stress (Webb *et al.*, 2008). With the decline of catecholamine levels in blood the number of lymphocytes in the blood falls as well (Schedlowski *et al.*, 1993, 1996). For example 60–120 minutes after finishing an acute bout of exercise with a clear secretion of adrenaline or after adrenaline infusions for 30–60 minutes, lymphopenia (low levels of lymphocytes) occurs in blood. Simultaneously, in parallel with the decrease of the lymphocyte subsets the counts of the neutrophil granulocytes are seen to rise (Gader and Cash, 1975; Crary *et al.*, 1983; Conlon *et al.*, 1988; Kappel *et al.*, 1991; Gabriel, 2000). The further stress hormone cortisol has been found to be responsible for the initiation of the lymphopenia and therefore the decrease of the number of NK cells in blood, the increase in the neutrophils and the reduction of the catecholamine (Shinkai *et al.*, 1996; Tonnesen *et al.*, 1987).

In conclusion, the immune system responds to the secretion of catecholamines immediately, almost independently of the kind of stressor. Depending on the concentration of catecholamines and the duration of the secretion, immune functions are controversially influenced; normally being suppressed.

Summary

The sympathetic branch of the ANS uses mainly catecholamines for signalling, they thus orchestrate numerous functions in the human body. The catecholamines are involved in almost all systems of energy demand as well as in multiple physiological situations such as illness, pain, hypoxia and hypoglycaemia, but they also play a major role in the response to psychological stimuli. The responsiveness of the ANS and thus the responsiveness of the secretion of catecholamines is under influence of age, gender, but also exercise intensity and duration. Research also shows that depending on intensity and duration, exercise leads to adaptive processes in the responsiveness of ANS and catecholamine secretion. Thus, in a psychoneuroendocrinology of sport and exercise both catecholamines and the role of exercise or physical fitness are important for the interpretation of psychobiological processes.

Nevertheless, inconsistent results produced by studies on adaptive processes, age, gender or exercise reflect that circadian rhythms, training status, psychosocial stressors as well as quantification methods of catecholamines and their metabolites are critical factors in the interpretation of results. Therefore, it is a considerable challenge to combine the various disciplines of biology, psychology and sports science to a psychoneuroendocrinology of sport and exercise. It is suggested that an integration of catecholamine research into the other orientations in sport psychology will allow, for example, research on the improvement of physical capacity by adaptive psychological intervention programmes or the use of exercise programmes as intervention models to change psychological behaviour.

References

Ader, R., Cohen, N. and Felten, D. (1995). Psychoneuroimmunology: Interactions between the nervous system and the immune system. *Lancet*, 345, 99–103.

Ahlborg, B. and Ahlborg, G. (1970). Exercise leukocytosis with and without beta-adrenergic blockade. *Acta Medica Scandinavica*, 187, 241–246.

Arner, P. (2005). Human fat cell lipolysis: biochemistry, regulation and clinical role. Best practice and research. *Clinical Endocrinology and Metabolism*, 19, 471–482.

Benschop, R. J., Nijkamp, F. P., Ballieux, R. E. and Heijnen, C. J. (1994). The effects of beta-adrenoceptor stimulation on adhesion of human natural killer cells to cultured endothelium. *British Journal of Pharmacology*, 113, 1311–1316.

Benschop, R. J., Oostveen, F. G., Heijnen, C. J. and Ballieux, R. E. (1993). Beta 2-adrenergic stimulation causes detachment of natural killer cells from cultured endothelium. *European Journal of Immunology*, 23, 3242–3247.

Benschop, R. J., Rodriguez-Feuerhahn, M. and Schedlowski, M. (1996). Catecholamine-induced leukocytosis: early observations, current research, and future directions. *Brain, Behavior and Immunity*, 10, 77–91.

Berczi, I. (1997). Pituitary hormones and immune function. *Acta Paediatrica Suppl*, 423, 70–75.

Berczi, I., Quintanar-Stephano, A. and Kovacs, K. (2009). Neuroimmune regulation in immunocompetence, acute illness, and healing. *Annals of the New York Academy of Sciences*, 1153, 220–239.

Besedovsky, H. O. and Del Rey, A. (1996). *Das immuno-neuroendokrine netzwerk [the immuno-neuroendocrine network]*. Heidelberg, Berlin: Spektrum.

Blomqvist, C. G., Lewis, S. F., Taylor, W. F. and Graham, R. M. (1981). Similarity of the hemodynamic responses to static and dynamic exercise of small muscle groups. *Circulation Research*, 48, 87–92.

Bloom, S. R., Johnson, R. H., Park, D. M., Rennie, M. J. and Sulaiman, W. R. (1976). Differences in the metabolic and hormonal response to exercise between racing cyclists and untrained individuals. *Journal of Physiology*, 258, 1–18.

Boutcher, S. H. and Hamer, M. (2006). Psychobiological reactivity, physical activity, and cardiovascular health. In E. Acevedo and P. Ekkekakis (eds), *Psychobiology of Physical Activity* (pp. 161–176). Champaign, IL: Human Kinetics.

Bremner, J. D., Krystal, J. H., Southwick, S. M. and Charney, D. S. (1996). Noradrenergic mechanisms in stress and anxiety: Ii. Clinical studies. *Synapse*, 23, 39–51.

Brohee, D., Vanhaeverbeek, M., Kennes, B. and Neve, P. (1990). Leukocyte and lymphocyte subsets after a short pharmacological stress by intravenous epinephrine and hydrocortisone in healthy humans. *International Journal of Neuroscience*, 53, 53–62.

Brosnan, J. T. (2003). Interorgan amino acid transport and its regulation. *Journal of Nutrition*, 133, 2068S–2072S.

Burns, A. M., Keogan, M., Donaldson, M., Brown, D. L. and Park, G. R. (1997). Effects of inotropes on human leucocyte numbers, neutrophil function and lymphocyte subtypes. *British Journal of Anaesthetics*, 78, 530–535.

Cheitlin, M. D. (2003). Cardiovascular physiology-changes with aging. *American Journal of Geriatric Cardiology*, 12, 9–13.

Christensen, N. J. and Brandsborg, O. (1973). The relationship between plasma catecholamine concentration and pulse rate during exercise and standing. *European Journal of Clinical Investigation*, 3, 299–306.

Chwalbinska-Moneta, J., Kruk, B., Nazar, K., Krzeminski, K., Kaciuba-Uscilko, H. and

Ziemba, A. (2005). Early effects of short-term endurance training on hormonal responses to graded exercise. *Journal of Physiology and Pharmacology*, 56, 87–99.

Cohen, C. I. (2002). Poverty, social problems, and serious mental illness. *Psychiatric Services*, 53, 899–900.

Conlon, P. D., Ogunbiyi, P. O., Black, W. D. and Eyre, P. (1988). Beta-adrenergic receptor function and oxygen radical production in bovine pulmonary alveolar macrophages. *Canadian Journal of Physiology and Pharmacology*, 66, 1538–1541.

Crary, B., Borysenko, M., Sutherland, D. C., Kutz, I., Borysenko, J. Z. and Benson, H. (1983). Decrease in mitogen responsiveness of mononuclear cells from peripheral blood after epinephrine administration in humans. *Journal of Immunology*, 130, 694–697.

Crews, D. J. and Landers, D. M. (1987). A meta-analytic review of aerobic fitness and reactivity to psychosocial stressors. *Medicine and Science in Sports and Exercise*, 19, 114–120.

Dantzer, R. and Kelley, K. W. (1989). Stress and immunity: an integrated view of relationships between the brain and the immune system. *Life Sciences*, 44, 1995–2008.

Davis, J. M., Albert, J. D., Tracy, K. J., *et al.* (1991). Increased neutrophil mobilization and decreased chemotaxis during cortisol and epinephrine infusions. *Journal of Trauma*, 31, 725–731; discussion 731–722.

Delanghe, J., De Slypere, J. P., De Buyzere, M., Robbrecht, J., Wieme, R. and Vermeulen, A. (1989). Normal reference values for creatine, creatinine, and carnitine are lower in vegetarians. *Clinical Chemistry*, 35, 1802–1803.

Delves, P. J., Martin, S. J., Burton, D. R. and Roitt, I. M. (2011). *Roitt's Essential Immunology*, 12th edn. Chichester: Wiley-Blackwell.

Dimsdale, J. E. and Moss, J. (1980). Short-term catecholamine response to psychological stress. *Psychosomatic Medicine*, 42, 493–497.

Dohrenwend, B. S. and Dohrenwend, B. P. (1970). *Class and Race as Status-related Sources of Stress*. Chicago: Aldine.

Drebing, C. J., Freedman, R., Waldo, M. and Gerhardt, G. A. (1989). Unconjugated methoxylated catecholamine metabolites in human saliva. Quantitation methodology and comparison with plasma levels. *Biomedical Chromatography*, 3, 217–220.

Eisenhofer, G., Kopin, I. J. and Goldstein, D. S. (2004). Catecholamine metabolism: a contemporary view with implications for physiology and medicine. *Pharmacological Reviews*, 56, 331–349.

Ferenčík, M., Rovenský, J., Mat'ha, V. and Herold, M. (2006). *Kompendium der Immunologie. Grundlagen und Klinik [Compendium Immunology. Foundations and Clinical Aspects]*. Wien: Springer Verlag.

Flaa, A., Ekeberg, O., Kjeldsen, S. and Rostrup, M. (2007). Personality may influence reactivity to stress. *BioPsychoSocial Medicine*, 1, 5.

Forsman, L. and Lundberg, U. (1982). Consistency in catecholamine and cortisol excretion in males and females. *Pharmacology Biochemistry and Behavior*, 17, 555–562.

Frankenhaeuser, M. (1971). Behavior and circulating catecholamines. *Brain Research*, 31, 241–262.

Frankenhaeuser, M. (ed.). (1975). *Experimental Approaches to the Study of Catecholamines and Emotion*. New York: Raven.

Frankenhaeuser, M. (1991). The psychophysiology of workload, stress, and health: Comparison between the sexes. *Annals of Behavioral Medicine*, 13, 197–205.

Frankenhaeuser, M., Sterky, K. and Jaerpe, G. (1962). Psychophysiological relations in habituation to gravitation stress. *Perceptual Motor Skills*, 15, 63–72.

French, E. B., Steel, C. M. and Aitchison, W. R. (1971). Studies on adrenaline-induced leucocytosis in normal man. II. The effects of alpha and beta adrenergic blocking agents. *British Journal of Haematology*, 21, 423–428.

Friedmann, B. and Kindermann, W. (1989). Energy metabolism and regulatory hormones in women and men during endurance exercise. *European Journal of Applied Physiology and Occupational Physiology*, 59, 1–9.

Funkenstein, D. H. (1956). Nor-epinephrine-like and epinephrine-like substances in relation to human behavior. *Journal of Nervous and Mental Disease*, 124, 58–68.

Gabriel, H. (2000). *Sport und Immunsystem – Modulationen und Adaptionen der Immunität Durch Belastung und Training [Sport and Immune System – Modulations and Adaptations through Strain and Train].* Schorndorf: Karl Hofmann.

Gader, A. M. and Cash, J. D. (1975). The effect of adrenaline, noradrenaline, isoprenaline and salbutamol on the resting levels of white blood cells in man. *Scandinavian Journal of Haematology*, 14, 5–10.

Galbo, H. (1983). *Hormonal and Metabolic Adaptation to Exercise.* New York: Thieme-Stratton.

Galbo, H., Holst, J. J. and Christensen, N. J. (1975). Glucagon and plasma catecholamine responses to graded and prolonged exercise in man. *Journal of Applied Physiology*, 38, 70–76.

Garcia-Sainz, J. A., Vazquez-Prado, J. and Villalobos-Molina, R. (1999). Alpha 1-adrenoceptors: subtypes, signaling, and roles in health and disease. *Archives of Medical Research*, 30, 449–458.

Garruti, G., Cotecchia, S., Giampetruzzi, F., Giorgino, F. and Giorgino, R. (2008). Neuroendocrine deregulation of food intake, adipose tissue and the gastrointestinal system in obesity and metabolic syndrome. *Journal of Gastrointestinal and Liver Diseases*, 17, 193–198.

Goldberger, L. (1993). Sensory deprivation and overload. In L. Goldberger and S. Breznitz (eds), *Handbook of Stress*, 2nd edn. (pp. 333–341). New York: Free Press.

Guezennec, Y., Leger, L., Lhoste, F., Aymonod, M. and Pesquies, P. C. (1986). Hormone and metabolite response to weight-lifting training sessions. *International Journal of Sports Medicine*, 7, 100–105.

Guezennec, C. Y., Oliver, C., Lienhard, F., Seyfried, D., Huet, F. and Pesce, G. (1992). Hormonal and metabolic response to a pistol-shooting competition. *Science and Sports*, 7, 27–32.

Hansen, A. M., Larsen, A. D., Rugulies, R., Garde, A. H. and Knudsen, L. E. (2009). A review of the effect of the psychosocial working environment on physiological changes in blood and urine. *Basic and Clinical Pharmacology and Toxicology*, 105, 73–83.

Harden, R. N., Rudin, N. J., Bruehl, S., Kee, W., Parikh, D. K., Kooch, J. and Gracely, R. H. (2004). Increased systemic catecholamines in complex regional pain syndrome and relationship to psychological factors: a pilot study. *Anesthesia and Analgesia*, 99, 1478–1485.

Harte, J. L. and Eifert, G. H. (1995). The effects of running, environment, and attentional focus on athletes' catecholamine and cortisol levels and mood. *Psychophysiology*, 32, 49–54.

Hellstrand, K., Hermodsson, S. and Strannegard, O. (1985). Evidence for a beta-adrenoceptor-mediated regulation of human natural killer cells. *Journal of Immunology*, 134, 4095–4099.

Hjemdahl, P., Freyschuss, U. and Juhlin-Dannfelt, A. (eds). (1986). *Plasma Catecholamines and Mental Stress.* Copenhagen: Munksgaard.

Holmes, D. S. (1993). Aerobic fitness and the response to psychological stress. In

P. Seraganian (ed.), *Exercise Psychology: the Influence of Physical Exercise on Psychological Processes* (pp. 39–63). New York: Wiley.

Horton, T. J., Pagliassotti, M. J., Hobbs, K. and Hill, J. O. (1998). Fuel metabolism in men and women during and after long-duration exercise. *Journal of Applied Physiology*, 85, 1823–1832.

Ingemarsson, I. (2003). Gender aspects of preterm birth. *BJOG: International Journal of Obstetrics and Gynaecology*, 110 (Suppl 20), 34–38.

Irwin, M., Thompson, J., Miller, C., Gillin, J. C. and Ziegler, M. (1999). Effects of sleep and sleep deprivation on catecholamine and interleukin-2 levels in humans: clinical implications. *Journal of Clinical Endocrinology and Metabolism*, 84, 1979–1985.

Jackson, E. M. and Dishman, R. K. (2006). Cardiorespiratory fitness and laboratory stress: a meta-regression analysis. *Psychophysiology*, 43, 57–72.

James, G. D., Crews, D. E. and Pearson, J. (1989). Catecholamines and stress. In M.A. Little and J.D. Haas (eds), *Human Population Biology: A Transdisciplinary Science* (pp. 280–295). Oxford: Oxford University Press.

Janeway, C. A. and Travers, P. (1995). *Immunologie*. Heidelberg: Spektrum.

Joh, T. H. and Hwang, O. (1987). Dopamine beta-hydroxylase: biochemistry and molecular biology. *Annals of the New York Academy of Sciences*, 493, 342–350.

Jones, G. (2008). Caffeine and other sympathomimetic stimulants: modes of action and effects on sports performance. *Essays in Biochemistry*, 44, 109–123.

Jörgensen, L. S., Bönlökke, L. and Christensen, N. J. (1985). Plasma adrenaline and noradrenaline during mental stress and isometric exercise in man. The role of arterial sampling. *Scandinavian Journal of Clinical and Laboratory Investigation*, 45, 447–452.

Juma, A. H., Ardawi, M. S., Baksh, T. M. and Serafi, A. A. (1991). Alterations in thyroid hormones, cortisol, and catecholamine concentration in patients after orthopedic surgery. *Journal of Surgical Research*, 50, 129–134.

Kappel, M., Tvede, N., Galbo, H., *et al.* (1991). Evidence that the effect of physical exercise on NK cell activity is mediated by epinephrine. *Journal of Applied Physiology*, 70, 2530–2534.

Kappel, M., Poulsen, T. D., Galbo, H. and Pedersen, B. K. (1998). Effects of elevated plasma noradrenaline concentration on the immune system in humans. *European Journal of Applied Physiology and Occupational Physiology*, 79, 93–98.

Kennedy, B., Dillon, E., Mills, P. J. and Ziegler, M. G. (2001). Catecholamines in human saliva. *Life Sciences*, 69, 87–99.

Khan, M. M., Sansoni, P., Silverman, E. D., Engleman, E. G. and Melmon, K. L. (1986). Beta-adrenergic receptors on human suppressor, helper, and cytolytic lymphocytes. *Biochemical Pharmacology*, 35, 1137–1142.

Kjaer, M. (1998). Adrenal medulla and exercise training. *European Journal of Applied Physiology and Occupational Physiology*, 77, 195–199.

Kjaer, M., Secher, N. H. and Galbo, H. (1987). Physical stress and catecholamine release. *Bailliere's Clinical Endocrinology and Metabolism*, 1, 279–298.

Kjaer, M., Bangsbo, J., Lortie, G. and Galbo, H. (1988). Hormonal response to exercise in humans: influence of hypoxia and physical training. *American Journal of Physiology*, 254, R197–203.

Kohrt, W. M., Spina, R. J., Ehsani, A. A., Cryer, P. E. and Holloszy, J. O. (1993). Effects of age, adiposity, and fitness level on plasma catecholamine responses to standing and exercise. *Journal of Applied Physiology*, 75, 1828–1835.

Kvetnansky, R., Sabban, E. L. and Palkovits, M. (2009). Catecholaminergic systems in stress: structural and molecular genetic approaches. *Physiological Reviews*, 89, 535–606.

Lambert, W. W., MacEvoy, B., Klackenberg-Larsson, I., Karlberg, P. and Karlberg, J. (1987). The relation of stress hormone excretion to type a behavior and to health. *Journal of Human Stress*, 13, 128–135.

Lazarus, R. S. and Folkman, S. (1984). *Psychological Stress and the Coping Process*. New York: Springer.

Li, G. Y., Ueki, H., Yamamoto, Y. and Yamada, S. (2006). Association between the scores on the general health questionnaire-28 and the saliva levels of 3-methoxy-4-hydroxy-phenylglycol in normal volunteers. *Biological Psychology*, 73, 209–211.

Loeper, M. and Crouzon, O. (1904). L'action de l'adrénaline sur le sang. *Archives de Médecine Expérimentale et D'anatomie Pathologique*, 16, 83–108.

Lub, M., van Kooyk, Y. and Figdor, C. G. (1995). Ins and outs of lfa-1. *Immunology Today*, 16, 479–483.

Maisel, A. S., Fowler, P., Rearden, A., Motulsky, H. J. and Michel, M. C. (1989). A new method for isolation of human lymphocyte subsets reveals differential regulation of beta-adrenergic receptors by terbutaline treatment. *Clinical Pharmacology and Therapeutics*, 46, 429–439.

Malarkey, W. B. and Mills, P. J. (2007). Endocrinology: the active partner in PNI research. *Brain, Behavior, and Immunity*, 21, 161–168.

Mason, J. W. (1968). A review of psychoendocrine research on the sympathetic-adrenal medullary system. *Psychosomatic Medicine*, 30 (Suppl), 631–653.

McCrimmon, D. R., Cunningham, D. A., Rechnitzer, P. A. and Griffiths, J. (1976). Effect of training on plasma catecholamines in post myocardial infarction patients. *Medicine and Science in Sports*, 8, 152–156.

Michelotti, G. A., Price, D. T. and Schwinn, D. A. (2000). Alpha 1-adrenergic receptor regulation: basic science and clinical implications. *Pharmacology and Therapeutics*, 88, 281–309.

Mond, J. J., Vos, Q., Lees, A. and Snapper, C. M. (1995). T cell independent antigens. *Current Opinion in Immunology*, 7, 349–354.

Motulsky, H. J. and Insel, P. A. (1982). Adrenergic receptors in man: direct identification, physiologic regulation, and clinical alterations. *New England Journal of Medicine*, 307, 18–29.

Mougios, V. (2006). *Exercise Biochemistry*. Champaign, IL: Human Kinetics.

Muir, A. L., Cruz, M., Martin, B. A., Thommasen, H., Belzberg, A. and Hogg, J. C. (1984). Leukocyte kinetics in the human lung: role of exercise and catecholamines. *Journal of Applied Physiology*, 57, 711–719.

Murphy, K. M., Travers, P. and Walport, M. (2009). *Janeway's Immunobiology*, 7th edn. New York: Garland Science.

Netter, P., Vogel, W. and Rammsayer, T. (1994). Extraversion as a modifying factor in catecholamine and behavioral responses to ethanol. *Psychopharmacology*, 115, 206–212.

Nordin, C. (2010). The case for hypoglycaemia as a proarrhythmic event: Basic and clinical evidence. *Diabetologia*, 53, 1552–1561.

Oeltmann, T., Carson, R., Shannon, J. R., Ketch, T. and Robertson, D. (2004). Assessment of o-methylated catecholamine levels in plasma and urine for diagnosis of autonomic disorders. *Autonomic Neuroscience: Basic and Clinical*, 116, 1–10.

Okamura, H., Tsuda, A., Yajima, J., *et al.* (2010). Short sleeping time and psychobiological responses to acute stress. *International Journal of Psychophysiology*, 78, 209–214.

Pacak, K. and Palkovits, M. (2001). Stressor specificity of central neuroendocrine responses: implications for stress-related disorders. *Endocrine Reviews*, 22, 502–548.

Pereira, S. B., Gava, I. A., Giro, C. and Mesquita, E. T. (2010). Adrenergic receptor poly-morphisms in heart failure: what can genetics explain? *Arquivos Brasileiros de Cardiologia*, 94, 841–849.

Péronnet, F., Massicotte, D., Paquet, J., Brisson, G. and de Champlain, J. (1989). Blood pressure and plasma catecholamine responses to various challenges during exercise-recovery in man. *European Journal of Applied Physiology and Occupational Physiology*, 58, 551–555.

Philipson, L. H. (2002). Beta-agonists and metabolism. *Journal of Allergy and Clinical Immunology*, 110, S313–317.

Purves, D., Augustine, G. J., Fitzpatrick, D., *et al.* (2007). *Neuroscience*, 4th edn. Sunderland, MA: Sinauer Associates.

Rabin, B. S., Moyna, N. M., Kusnecov, A., Zhou, D. and Shurin, M. R. (1996). Neuroendocrine effects on immunity. In L. Hoffman-Goetz (ed.), *Exercise and Immune Function*. Boca Raton, FL: CRC Press.

Roitt, I. M., Brostoff, J. and Male, D.K. (1995). *Kurzes Lehrbuch der Immunologie*, 3rd edn. Stuttgart: Thieme.

Ronsen, O., Haug, E., Pedersen, B. K. and Bahr, R. (2001). Increased neuroendocrine response to a repeated bout of endurance exercise. *Medicine and Science in Sports and Exercise*, 33, 568–575.

Rosano, T. G., Swift, T. A. and Hayes, L. W. (1991). Advances in catecholamine and metabolite measurements for diagnosis of pheochromocytoma. *Clinical Chemistry*, 37, 1854–1867.

Roy, A., De Jong, J. and Linnoila, M. (1989). Extraversion in pathological gamblers. Correlates with indexes of noradrenergic function. *Archives of General Psychiatry*, 46, 679–681.

Salmon, P. (1992). Psychological factors in surgical stress: implications for management. *Clinical Psychology Review*, 12, 681–704.

Schedlowski, M., Falk, A., Rohne, A., *et al.* (1993). Catecholamines induce alterations of distribution and activity of human NK cells. *Journal of Clinical Immunology*, 13, 344–351.

Schedlowski, M., Hosch, W., Oberbeck, R., *et al.* (1996). Catecholamines modulate human nk cell circulation and function via spleen-independent beta 2-adrenergic mechanisms. *Journal of Immunology*, 156, 93–99.

Schmidt, R. F., Lang, F. and Heckmann, M. (eds). (2007). *Physiologie des Menschen*. Heidelberg: Springer.

Schuler, J. L. and O'Brien, W. H. (1997). Cardiovascular recovery from stress and hypertension risk factors: a meta-analytic review. *Psychophysiology*, 34, 649–659.

Schulz, T. (2002). *Ausdauersport und Immunsystem – Langzeiteffekte eines Leistungstrainings auf das Zelluläre Immunsystem bei Radsportlern [Endurance Training and Immune System – Long-term Effects of Training on the Cellular Immune System in Cyclists]*. Köln: Sport and Buch Strauß.

Seals, D. R. and Esler, M. D. (2000). Human ageing and the sympathoadrenal system. *Journal of Physiology*, 528, 407–417.

Segerstrom, S. C. and Miller, G. E. (2004). Psychological stress and the human immune system: a meta-analytic study of 30 years of inquiry. *Psychological Bulletin*, 130, 601–630.

Shepard, R. J. (2003). Adhesion molecules, catecholamine and leucocyte redistribution during and following exercise. *Sports Medicine*, 33, 261–284.

Sherman, D. K., Bunyan, D. P., Creswell, J. D. and Jaremka, L. M. (2009). Psychological vulnerability and stress: the effects of self-affirmation on sympathetic nervous system responses to naturalistic stressors. *Health Psychology*, 28, 554–562.

Shinkai, S., Watanabe, S., Asai, H. and Shek, P. N. (1996). Cortisol response to exercise and post-exercise suppression of blood lymphocyte subset counts. *International Journal of Sports Medicine*, 17, 597–603.

Sokolov, E. I., Podachin, V. P. and Belova, E. V. (1983). *Emotional Stress and Cardiovascular Response*. Moscow: Mir.

Sothmann, M. S. (2006). The cross-stressor adaptation hypothesis and exercise training. In E.O. Acevedo and P. Ekkekakis (eds), *Psychobiology of Physical Activity* (pp. 149–160). Champaign, IL: Human Kinetics.

Sothmann, M. S., Horn, T. S., Hart, B. A. and Gustafson, A. B. (1987). Comparison of discrete cardiovascular fitness groups on plasma catecholamine and selected behavioral responses to psychological stress. *Psychophysiology*, 24, 47–54.

Sothmann, M. S., Hart, B. A. and Horn, T. S. (1991). Plasma catecholamine response to acute psychological stress in humans: relation to aerobic fitness and exercise training. *Medicine and Science in Sports and Exercise*, 23, 860–867.

Sothmann, M. S., Hart, B. A. and Horn, T. S. (1992). Sympathetic nervous system and behavioral responses to stress following exercise training. *Physiology and Behavior*, 51, 1097–1103.

Souza-Moreira, L., Campos-Salinas, J., Caro, M. and Gonzalez-Rey, E. (2011). Neuropeptides as pleiotropic modulators of the immune response. *Neuroendocrinology*, 94, 89–100.

Stock, C., Zimmermann, E. and Teuchert-Noodt, G. (1993). Effect of examination stress on sympathetic activity and β-adrenergic receptors. *Journal of Psychophysiology*, 7, 310–307.

Suzuki, K., Totsuka, M., Nakaji, S., Yamada, M., Kudoh, S., Liu, Q., and Sato, K. (1999). Endurance exercise causes interaction among stress hormones, cytokines, neutrophil dynamics, and muscle damage. *Journal of Applied Physiology*, 87, 1360–1367.

Taggart, P. and Carruthers, M. (1971). Endogenous hyperlipidaemia induced by emotional stress of racing driving. *Lancet*, 1, 363–366.

Taylor, A. H. (2000). Physical activity, anxiety and stress. In S. J. H. Biddle, K. R. Fox and S. H. Boutcher (eds), *Physical Activity and Psychological Well-being* (pp. 10–45). London: Routledge.

Thomas, G. D. (2011). Neural control of the circulation. *Advances in Physiology Education*, 35, 28–32.

Tonnesen, E., Christensen, N. J. and Brinklov, M. M. (1987). Natural killer cell activity during cortisol and adrenaline infusion in healthy volunteers. *European Journal of Clinical Investigation*, 17, 497–503.

van Doornen, L. J. and van Blokland, R. W. (1989). The relation of type a behavior and vital exhaustion with physiological reactions to real life stress. *Journal of Psychosomatic Research*, 33, 715–725.

van Tits, L. J. and Graafsma, S. J. (1991). Stress influences cd4+ lymphocyte counts. *Immunology Letters*, 30, 141–142.

Vecht, R. J., Graham, G. W. and Sever, P. S. (1978). Plasma noradrenaline concentrations during isometric exercise. *British Heart Journal*, 40, 1216–1220.

Webb, H. E., Weldy, M. L., Fabianke-Kadue, E. C., Orndorff, G. R., Kamimori, G. H. and Acevedo, E. O. (2008). Psychological stress during exercise: cardiorespiratory and hormonal responses. *European Journal of Applied Physiology*, 104, 973–981.

Weise, M., Eisenhofer, G. and Merke, D. P. (2002). Pubertal and gender-related changes in the sympathoadrenal system in healthy children. *Journal of Clinical Endocrinology and Metabolism*, 87, 5038–5043.

Wheatley, K., Creed, M. and Mellor, A. (2011). Haematological changes at altitude. *Journal of the Royal Army Medical Corps*, 157, 38–42.

Wolthers, B. G., Kema, I. P., Volmer, M., Wesemann, R., Westermann, J. and Manz, B. (1997). Evaluation of urinary metanephrine and normetanephrine enzyme immunoassay (elisa) kits by comparison with isotope dilution mass spectrometry. *Clinical Chemistry*, 43, 114–120.

Wood, J. D. (1999). Neurotransmission at the interface of sympathetic and enteric divisions of the autonomic nervous system. *Chinese Journal of Physiology*, 42, 201–210.

Zouhal, H., Jacob, C., Delamarche, P. and Gratas-Delamarche, A. (2008). Catecholamines and the effects of exercise, training and gender. *Sports Medicine*, 38, 401–423.

6   Salivary alpha-amylase

Jana Strahler

Salivary measures are becoming increasingly important in the assessment of physiological biomarkers in sport and exercise. Hormones such as cortisol or dehydroepiandrosterone can be easily measured in saliva as meaningful markers for various exercise and training-related processes in the body. The salivary enzyme alpha-amylase (sAA) has been suggested to reflect stress-related changes in the body (e.g. Rohleder *et al.*, 2004). Its secretion is known to be elicited by activation of the autonomic nervous system which controls the salivary glands. This chapter will provide an overview of the use of sAA as a biomarker reflecting (stress) responses to physical strain and the competitive demands in sport (see also Table 6.5).

Physiology and mechanisms

Secretion

Salivary alpha-amylase is the most important and abundant protein in saliva. It constitutes about 10% of overall salivary protein content (Witt, 2006). In humans, total sAA production is estimated to be 1.5 g per day, 60% of which is released by the pancreas and 40% by salivary glands, mainly the parotid glands. This enzyme is known to be mainly involved in the initiation of the digestion of starch in the oral cavity. Furthermore, sAA has also been shown to have an important antibacterial function.

Amylase is primarily produced by acinar cells. Acinar cells are innervated by both the sympathetic and the parasympathetic branches of the autonomic nervous system (ANS). Noradrenaline released from sympathetic neurons binds to both alpha- and beta-adrenergic receptors on the acinar cell, leading to an increase in the second messenger cyclic adenosine monophosphate (cAMP) and thus increasing salivary protein secretion. Studies using blocking or stimulating pharmacological agents or electrical stimuli have helped us to understand the secretory mechanisms of sAA release. These studies indicate that beta-adrenergic mechanisms are the main contributing factor in sAA secretion.

One of the first studies suggesting sAA as a marker of sympathetic activity was conducted by Speirs and colleagues (Speirs *et al.*, 1974). The authors either administered the beta-adrenergic agonist isoprenaline or the beta-adrenergic blocker propranolol or they immersed subjects in cold water (4–5°C), causing an acute autonomic response. Cold water and isoprenaline increased sAA in parotid saliva, while propanolol led to a reduction in sAA. This latter finding was confirmed by more recent studies, revealing that propranolol attenuates stress-induced sAA increases (van Stegeren *et al.*, 2006). Ehlert and colleagues (2006) examined the effect of yohimbine hydrochloride, an alpha$_2$-adrenergic receptor antagonist, on sAA release. As expected, larger increases in sAA activity were found in the yohimbine challenge condition than in the control group. These findings suggest that changes in sAA might be regarded as an indirect indicator of changes in autonomic activation. Furthermore, there is a well-known effect of mechanical and gustatory stimulation on salivary amylase secretion which will be discussed below.

Short-term regulation

As we have learned, the release of sAA is governed by activation of the ANS. An increase in sAA may thus be expected during periods of physiological and psychological stress (i.e. when autonomic activation is high). Various studies have reported increased sAA activity after various acute stressors. Salivary alpha-amylase has been shown to be a correlate of adrenergic reactivity to physiological stress conditions (Chatterton *et al.*, 1996) and psychosocial stress (e.g. Rohleder *et al.*, 2004). The enzyme was also shown to increase during simulated critical incident scenarios in police officers, which therefore mimics occupational stress (Groer *et al.*, 2010). Furthermore, the blocking effects of beta-adrenergic antagonists on sAA concentrations in human saliva clearly indicate that sAA is a measure of autonomic activity (Speirs *et al.*, 1974; van Stegeren *et al.*, 2006).

Table 6.1 provides an overview of the different protocols that are used to stimulate sAA. Almost uniformly, these tests have resulted in sAA increases immediately after the stressor and rapidly declining values thereafter. This is in contrast to the response pattern of salivary cortisol, a measure of the activity of the hypothalamic–pituitary–adrenocortical (HPA) axis (see Chapter 3), which peaks about 20 minutes post-stressor. Amylase therefore provides a useful, non-invasive, highly sensitive parameter reflecting fast autonomic changes.

Long-term regulation

Analysing salivary flow rate and protein content in whole saliva and stimulated parotid saliva from healthy women and men, Dawes was one of the first to show a significant diurnal rhythmicity of these measurements (Dawes, 1972). One of the first reviews on this issue (Ferguson *et al.*, 1973) summarized seven studies which also measured sAA. In this review, one study reported higher morning values of sAA, whereas four others reported higher afternoon values. These findings were replicated in other studies analysing stimulated and non-stimulated whole saliva

Table 6.1 Summary and selection of psycho(-social) and physiological stress protocols (see also Table 6.4) in amylase research

Study	Stressor	Design	Subjects	Results
Psycho(-social) stress protocols in general				
Gordis et al., 2008	Modified TSST	−45, −5, +1, +10, +20, +30 min	47 maltreated adolescents (21 ♀), 9–14 yrs 37 controls (19 ♀), 9–14 yrs	Amylase increase immediately post-stressor; 63.1% of youths showing increases greater than 10%; attenuated responses in maltreated youths.
Perroni et al., 2009	Simulated firefighting	pre, +30, +90 min	20 male firefighters, 32 ± 6 yrs	Amylase increase 174% above pre-test values.
Spinrad et al., 2009	Frustrating task	pre, +10, +40 min	84 preschoolers (41 ♀), ø 54 mo	47% of children at least 10% amylase increase; amylase reactivity related to dispositional anger, impulsivity, regulation, and externalizing problems (in girls).
Groer et al., 2010	Virtual critical incident scenario (chase)	pre, +10, +30 min	141 law enforcement volunteer officers (27 ♀), 22–64 yrs, ø 37 yrs	Amylase increase; association with IL-6 and IgA; positive correlation years of police experience and amylase.
Kang, 2010	Academic final test	−45, −30, −15, −1, +1, +15, +30 min	16 healthy female students, 21.8 ± 1.2 yrs 17 healthy controls (7 ♀), 20.3 ± 1.4 yrs	Amylase increase; amylase associated with other autonomic markers (plasma catecholamines, blood pressure, and heart rate), but only marginal.
McKay et al., 2010	Induction and intubation sequence in a patient simulator	−1, +1, +20 min	18 young nurse anaesthesia students (3 ♀; 6 low-, 6 moderate-, and 6 high-performing subjects)	Amylase increase independent of performance level (119% increase in low, 0.6% increase in moderate, 114% increase in high performers).
Rai and Kaur, 2011	21 days of 6° head-down tilt	Pre, end task, 1, 2, 3 wk	12 healthy men, ø 25 yrs	Steadily increasing amylase levels throughout the study.
(Competitive) physiological stress protocols				
Speirs et al., 1974	Cold water immersion (4–5°C); isoprenaline; propranolol	Baseline, 45–120 min following ingestion	6 subjects	Amylase increase due to cold water immersion and circulating isoprenaline (stimulant); reduction in amylase activity following propranolol (beta blocker).

Study	Intervention	Measurement times	Participants	Results
Pilardeau et al., 1990	Acute altitude hypoxia (2 days at 4350 m) + maximal exercise	Rest and immediately following maximal exercise	12 young adults (4 ♀), 35.5 ± 7 yrs	No effect of exercise performed in normoxia and hypoxia on saliva flow and amylase; acute hypoxia increased saliva flow rate but not amylase (descriptively decreased).
Calvo et al., 1997	Progressive treadmill test	Pre, at the end of each 5 min stage	20 healthy males (military training course), 21 ± 3 yrs	Positive association amylase and lactate (amylase as non-invasive marker of aerobic fitness); increase in amylase with intense exercise.
Li and Gleeson, 2004	Cycling at 60% Vo_{2max}	−10 min, after exercising for 1 h, 2 h, 1 and 2 h postexercise	8 healthy men	Amylase increase, independent of time of day; a 3 h rest enough to recover from previous strenuous exercise.
Kivlighan and Granger, 2006	Rowing ergometer competition	Pre, +20, +40 min	14 (4 ♀) varsity rowers, 17–31 yrs 28 (17 ♀) novice rowers, 17–31 yrs	156% amylase increase in response to the ergometer competition; amylase higher across the competition for varsity compared to novice rowers; positive association amylase and performance and interest in teambonding.
Chiodo et al., 2011	Taekwondo competition	Pre, end task, +30 min	16 youth athletes (6 ♀), 13–14 yrs	115% amylase increase at the end of match, within 30 minutes of recovery return to baseline level; no gender difference.
Strahler et al., 2011	Ballroom dancing competition	Pre, end first round, +30 min, 8 p.m.	32 younger dancer (18 ♀), 21.4 ± 4.0 yrs 37 senior dancer (17 ♀), 60.6 ± 7.8 yrs	Increase in amylase after the first round; higher response in senior dancers; no association amylase response and subjective stress experiences.

TSST, Trier Social Stress Test; Vo_{2max}, maximal oxygen consumption.

from healthy students (Jenzano *et al.*, 1987; Artino *et al.*, 1998; Rantonen and Meurman, 2000; Li and Gleeson, 2004) and from diabetic patients (Artino *et al.*, 1998). In contrast, Yamaguchi and colleagues (2006) did not observe significant changes over time in healthy male students when using a handheld electronic measurement device.

More recent studies using salivettes have found a pronounced daily profile of sAA activity which is characterized by a strong decrease in the morning and steadily increasing values throughout the day that peak in the late afternoon (e.g. Nater *et al.*, 2007). Among the few studies assessing full daily profiles, one study could not find this drop within the first 30 minutes after awakening (Michaud *et al.*, 2006). These authors also found no effect of noise (i.e. sleep disturbances) and sleeping at home vs. in the laboratory on morning sAA rhythms.

Determination and assessment

When measuring sAA activity, several methodological aspects have to be taken into account. Researchers have to decide which sampling method to take, how to store samples, which determination method to use and how to handle data statistically.

Sampling methods

One of the most commonly used techniques to collect stimulated whole saliva is through the use of oral swabs. This device mostly consists of a plastic vessel, a centrifugation tube and a cotton or synthetic swab. When assessing cortisol levels the use of oral swabs is currently viewed as the 'gold standard' (Kirschbaum and Hellhammer, 1999). Measuring sAA activity with this device might be confounded by stimulation of saliva flow. This is due to their short-term functionality in the digestion of starches. Salivary flow rate and composition are influenced by primary oral stimulation, such as chewing and food properties (Froehlich *et al.*, 1987; Mackie and Pangborn, 1990) and by alterations of parasympathetic nervous system activity (Anderson *et al.*, 1984; Garrett, 1987). Moreover, changes of sAA activity are a primary response to oral stimulation alone since oral stimulation effectively changes amylase secretion rate but not its concentration (Froehlich *et al.*, 1987; Mackie and Pangborn, 1990). Increased flow rate values parallel a higher sAA secretion rate, with more sAA being available for digestion while its concentration in saliva remains unaffected. As the parasympathetic nervous system is the primary mediator of salivary flow rate, acute stress-induced sympathetic activation and parasympathetic inhibition would decrease flow rate. Together with unchanged protein secretion from acinar cells this theoretically leads to higher protein concentrations without increased protein secretion per se. Rohleder and colleagues (2006) tested this hypothesis and found that stress-induced increases of sAA levels were correlated with increases of amylase output but not with flow rate. Furthermore, flow rate increased only when sampled by passive drooling but not when using salivettes. It was therefore concluded that salivettes are a valid sampling technique independent of the assessment of flow rate.

Just recently, Beltzer and colleagues (2010) compared different sampling techniques (microsponge cotton pledget, synthetic oral swab and passive drool), different collection point duration (1–5 minutes) and oral fluid type (whole non-stimulated, parotid, submandibular and sublingual saliva). In sum, since sAA is an enzyme directly produced in the salivary glands, the results highlight the importance of standardizing collection techniques and protocols to minimize unsystematic variation related to how, when and where saliva is collected. Furthermore, it was suggested that a chewing-stimulated increase of salivary flow leads to alterations of pH value and thereby to changes in enzymatic activity. To test this hypothesis, we carried out a study in which sample pH value was changed with hydrochloride or sodium hydroxide. Analyses revealed no difference between treated and untreated samples (all $t51 < 0.8$, $P < 0.44$). These data indicate that there is no alteration of sAA activity level after changing the pH value of the saliva sample (Strahler, unpublished data).

Storage of samples

Salivary alpha-amylase is classified as a relatively stable protein (Gasteiger *et al.*, 2005). Nevertheless, it is recommended to store samples at –20°C or lower temperatures if longer storage (up to 12 months) is planned (for an excellent review of methodological considerations see Rohleder and Nater, 2009). It was shown that sAA obtained with the help of salivettes remains stable following five days at room temperature, and five freeze–thaw cycles (O'Donnell *et al.*, 2009). In agreement with this, DeCaro (2008) reported no effect on sAA activity of storage at room temperature or 37°C for up to three weeks.

Determination method

Many techniques are available for analysing sAA, with enzyme kinetic methods being the most commonly used (see also Rohleder and Nater, 2009). This procedure quantifies alpha-amylase activity by measuring a specific substrate that is metabolized due to the enzymatic action of sAA. The resulting cleavage products can be measured spectrophotometrically, with the amount of sAA activity in the sample being directly proportional to the increase in absorbance.

Statistical handling

Different measures can be used to indicate sAA. The most common index of sAA activity is the determination of enzyme level per volume of saliva (enzyme units per milliliter, U/mL). However, this is only an indirect measure of sAA concentration and is defined as the amount of enzyme that catalyses the conversion of 1 μmol of substrate per minute. Therefore, total enzyme output in a fixed time interval is also often given as enzyme units per minute (U/min). Since the specific activity in relation to other salivary proteins may also be of interest, enzyme units per milligram protein (U/mg) is another index.

Values of sAA activity are typically positively skewed and more frequently demonstrate higher variability than, for example, salivary cortisol. Possible reasons for this phenomenon may lie in the fast responsiveness of sAA to psychological as well as physical or gustatory stimuli, as well as to variability in sampling techniques (e.g. duration of saliva accumulation). Using logarithmic or square root transformation can successfully restore normal distribution.

Subsequent analysis, vary depending on the research question and design. To capture acute sAA responses as well as recovery it is recommended to collect saliva at baseline, if possible also during the stressor, immediately after the intervention and frequently thereafter up to every 5 minutes until at least 30 minutes afterwards (e.g. mental stress test, competition). Calculating indices of sAA responses, researchers most often use simpler indices such as the delta score between baseline and post-intervention maximum as peak stress response. More complex indices are also used, such as the slope of the regression curve immediately post-intervention and later on, as a recovery index or the area under the curve with respect to increase (i.e. ignoring the distance from zero for all measurements and thereby emphasizing changes over time) (Pruessner *et al.*, 2003).

When measuring diurnal profiles of sAA activity, as discussed below, it is recommended to obtain several samples throughout the day relative to awakening. Due to strong diurnal variation, especially in the morning hours, samples should be collected at least 30 minutes after awakening, and frequently afterwards to cover the whole day until bedtime. Although a good stability of diurnal rhythm has been shown (Wolf *et al.*, 2008), diurnal profiles should be collected on at least two consecutive days. Traditionally, two different indices are calculated to assess basal sAA activity: the area under the curve with respect to ground (i.e. the overall diurnal output) and the slope of the profile. Furthermore, it is advisable to objectively control for compliance by using electronic monitors or personal digital assistants (PDAs) as well as objectively assessing wake-up time with the help of activity monitors.

Modulating factors influencing amylase (re-)activity

There are multiple factors that might influence sAA activity and are therefore in the focus of current research. This section will describe those factors with a special emphasis on sport psychology issues.

When investigating modulating factors of sAA activity, we have to differentiate between influences on acute alterations and determinants of basal values of this enzyme. As discussed above, sAA activity could be described as a fast-reacting physiological response (Nater *et al.*, 2005, 2006; Rohleder *et al.*, 2004, 2008). But it is not only acute changes that need to be mentioned, determinants having more lasting effects such as age, sex, smoking and physical fitness also influence acute sAA secretion as well as basal levels in general. In the following section, background and recent findings on methodological issues and potential factors influencing sAA measurement are summarized.

Age effects

Most studies of the acute stress-induced changes of sAA activity have been conducted with adult participants. Knowledge of younger age groups is rare and only few studies looked at older populations. With regard to younger age groups, a heel prick test in neonates did not result in significant increases in sAA (Schaffer *et al.*, 2008), and Davis and Granger (2009) reported sAA increases to a painful stressor in infants aged six and twelve months. Much more evidence exists for acute sAA responses in older children and adolescents. The results of these studies imply that adolescents respond with similar magnitudes as adults. To date, only one study has compared the responses of different age groups to a similar laboratory stress task. Higher pre-stress levels of sAA in children and attenuated sAA responses in children and older adults were found (Strahler *et al.*, 2010a). The only study assessing age effects on the responses of athletes to competition revealed higher sAA responses in senior ballroom dancers compared to younger ones (Strahler *et al.*, 2011).

The youngest age group in which basal sAA has been investigated were newborns. Studies found sAA levels to be very low to undetectable in this group and that they gradually increased to reach adult levels within the first three months of age (Sevenhuysen *et al.*, 1984). After that, amylase activity levels remained stable into older adulthood in stimulated as well as non-stimulated whole saliva (Ben-Aryeh *et al.*, 1990).

However, in all the studies described above, saliva was obtained at one single point in time; studies looking at diurnal changes of sAA activity are still rare. Pronounced changes of daily sAA activity have been found throughout a wide age range in children (Maldonado *et al.*, 2008; Wolf *et al.*, 2008), young adults (e.g. Nater *et al.*, 2007; Rohleder *et al.*, 2008) and older adults (Strahler *et al.*, 2010b). We were also able to show a pronounced daily profile at a heightened level in older adults (sympathetic overactivity). Examining a possible age effect on basal amylase in athletes, analyses showed flatter daily amylase slopes in younger dancers and attenuated amylase changes after awakening in younger male dancers, while the profiles of senior ballroom dancers showed the expected rhythm (Strahler *et al.*, 2010b).

In summary, while keeping the methodological limitations of some results in mind, acute stress responses are absent in newborns, can be measured in infants as young as six months, develop during childhood depending on the intervention, reach adult levels in adolescence and again attenuate in older adulthood. Furthermore the level of basal amylase activity changes over the lifespan, with higher values in older age groups. Reports of a possible age effect on amylase in athletes hints towards higher stress responses in older athletes, while the rhythms remain unaltered (Table 6.2).

Table 6.2 Summary of age effects on stress-induced and basal salivary α-amylase activity

Study	Measure/ stressor	Design	Subjects	Results
Acute stress responses				
Schaffer et al., 2008	Heel prick test	−10, +5, +20 min	18 small for gestational age (GA) neonates (12 ♀) 34 appropriate for GA neonates (18 ♀)	No group differences for amylase resting level; neonatal stress stimulus revealed similar response patterns.
Davis and Granger, 2009	Well-baby exam/ inoculation stress protocol	pre-test, +5, +10, +20 min	22 infants (11 ♀) 2 mo 19 infants (10 ♀) 6 mo 22 infants (11 ♀) 12 mo 22 infants (13 ♀) 24 mo	Older infants (24 mo) higher amylase levels; stress-related increases evident at 6 and 12 mo, but not at 2 or 24 mo of age.
Strahler et al., 2010a	TSST, TSST-C	−1, +1, +10, +20 min	62 children (30 females), 6–10 yrs 78 young adults (33 ♀), 20–31 yrs 74 older adults (37 ♀), 59–61 yrs	Higher amylase baseline in children; attenuated increase in children and older adults.
Strahler et al., 2011	Ballroom dancing competition	Pre, end first round, +30 min, 8 p.m.	32 younger dancer (18 ♀), 21.4 ± 4.0 yrs 37 senior dancer (17 ♀), 60.6 ± 7.8 yrs	Increase in amylase after the first round; higher response in senior dancers; no association amylase response and subjective stress experiences.
One-point basal measurements				
Hodge et al., 1983	Non-stimulated whole saliva	Basal amylase (9 a.m.–4 p.m.)	13 infants, 26–32 wk	Amylase increased with increasing age.
Sevenhuysen et al., 1984	Non-stimulated whole saliva	Basal amylase (1–6 p.m.)	29 infants, birth, 1, 2, 3, 4, and 5 mo ± 7 days	Low amylase activity at birth to 2/3 of adults by 3 months.
Aguirre et al., 1987	Stimulated parotid saliva	Basal amylase (8 a.m.–noon)	45 young adults, 20–39 yrs 40 middle-aged adults, 40–59 yrs 43 older adults, 60–84 yrs	No effect of age.

| Ben-Aryeh et al., 1990 | Non-stimulated whole saliva | Basal amylase (in the morning) | 25 infants (6 ♀), 7–11 mo; 28 toddlers (13 ♀), 2–3 yrs; 28 children (15 ♀), 6–8 yrs; 28 adolescents (14 ♀), 12–14 yrs; 27 adults (14 ♀), 25–63 yrs | Amylase very variable; differences between infants and toddlers; afterwards levels remained stable into adulthood. |

Diurnal profiles (more than two measurement timepoints)

Nater et al., 2007	Stimulated whole saliva	Amylase profile (waking, +30 min, +60 min, every hour to 8 p.m.)	76 healthy adults (44 ♀), 18–58 yrs, 26.7 ± 8.8 yrs	Linear increase in amylase attenuated by 0.6% with each year of age.
Wingenfeld et al., 2010	Stimulated whole saliva	Amylase profile (7 a.m., 11.30 a.m., 5.30 p.m., 8 p.m.)	215 nurses (168 ♀), 18–59 yrs	No effect of age, neither output nor slope.
Strahler et al., 2010b	Stimulated whole saliva	Amylase profile (waking, +30 min, 11 a.m., 3 p.m., 8 p.m.)	27 young dancers (15 ♀), 15–30 yrs; 26 young adults (12♀), 20–29 yrs; 31 older dancers (13 ♀), 49–75 yrs; 33 older adults (14 ♀), 51–75 yrs	Flattened daily amylase slope in younger dancers and older controls; higher overall amylase output in older adults; younger male dancers and older male controls lowest amylase change after awakening.

TSST/TSST-C, Trier Social Stress Test/Trier Social Stress Test for Children.

Gender effects

Many endocrine systems show a well-described sexual dimorphism, as for example the HPA axis (Kirschbaum *et al.*, 1999 see Chapter 3). Only a few studies have examined the possible effects of gonadal steroid changes (i.e. menstrual cycle or pregnancy) on the secretion of saliva and its components.

Studies investigating gender effects on acute sAA responses to stress have revealed no differences between men and women (e.g. van Stegeren *et al.*, 2008). This was true for sAA responses to multiple stress intervention including competition stress (see Table 6.3). Moreover, there seems to be no effect of hormonal status (i.e. of menstrual cycle) (Schoofs *et al.*, 2008). However, pregnancy may have a profound effect (Nierop *et al.*, 2006).

No sex differences in basal amylase activity have been reported so far. However, there is one recent study assessing the profiles of older adults and this study reported an effect of gender, with older men lacking the typical decrease in the morning. However, this age effect seems to be absent in athletes (Strahler *et al.*, 2010a).

Concerning the impact of steroid hormone status, current data do not support gender differences in basal and stress-induced sAA activity, and no effect of menstrual cycle phase has been recorded. In contrast, data regarding the impact of pregnancy remain inconclusive. Acute sAA responses were found to be attenuated in pregnant women. To the best of our knowledge, there have been no systematic studies examining acute stress-induced sAA changes in different phases of the menstrual cycle and little is known about differences between female and male athletes in this respect.

Lifestyle factors and health

When employing salivary measurements in studies in sport psychology, several exogenous factors need to be considered that may be associated with individual differences in salivary hormones and enzymes. The following sections describe major confounding variables of salivary alpha-amylase activity, including (1) lifestyle factors such as tobacco smoking, alcohol, caffeine, adiposity, food intake, and (2) factors associated with disease such as acute and chronic somatic and psychiatric diseases, and medical drugs.

Impact of smoking

It is known that nicotine activates the ANS (for a review see Adamopoulos *et al.*, 2008). Cigarette smoking should therefore be associated with increased sAA activity. However, the majority of studies reported that smoking is associated with decreased sAA activity after acute tobacco intake. Whether there is a difference between habitual smokers and non-smokers according to their sAA activity is another issue of interest. Up to date, only two studies have looked at this question. They found baseline levels to be lower in habitual smokers (Goi *et al.*,

Table 6.3 Summary of gender effects on stress-induced and basal salivary α-amylase activity

Study	Measure/stressor	Design	Subjects	Results
Acute stress responses				
Kivlighan and Granger, 2006	Rowing ergometer competition	Pre, +20, +40 min	14 (4 ♀) varsity rowers, 17–31 yrs 28 (17 ♀) novice rowers, 17–31 yrs	No main effect of gender on amylase in any phase of the competition.
Nierop et al., 2006	TSST	–20, –10, 0, +10, +20, +30, +40, +50, +60, +70, +80 min	30 second trimester ♀, 21–35 yrs 30 third trimester ♀, 21–35 yrs 30 non-pregnant ♀ in follicular phase, 21–37 yrs	Attenuated amylase increase in both pregnant groups compared to non-pregnant women.
Schoofs et al., 2008	Oral academic examination	–1, +1 min	40 undergraduate students (29 ♀, 18 OC users), 21.5 ± 0.3 yrs	No effect of gender and hormonal status.
van Stegeren et al., 2008	Cold pressure test	–30, 0, +10, +20, +60 min	80 healthy adults (21 ♂, 37 OC users, 22 non-OC), 20.7 ± 3.2 yrs	No effect of gender.
Strahler et al., 2010a	TSST, TSST-C	–1, +1, +10, +20 min	62 children (30 ♀), 6–10 yrs 78 young adults (33 ♀), 20–31 yrs 74 older adults (37 ♀), 59–61 yrs	No effect of gender.
Chiodo et al., 2011	Taekwondo competition	Pre, end task, +30 min	16 youth athletes (6 ♀), 13–14 yrs	No effect of gender.
Strahler et al., 2011	Ballroom dancing competition	Pre, end first round, +30 min, 8 p.m.	32 young dancers (18 ♀), 21.4 ± 4.0 yrs 37 senior dancers (17 ♀), 60.6 ± 7.8 yrs	No effect of gender.
One-point basal measurements				
Bhoola et al., 1978	Non-stimulated whole saliva	2 times morning and afternoon	220 girls, 14–18 yrs	No effect of menstrual cycle phase; amylase 2.5-fold higher in morning than in afternoon.

Table 6.3 Continued

Study	Measure/stressor	Design	Subjects	Results
D'Alessandro et al., 1989	Stimulated parotid saliva	Basal amylase (time not specified)	107 pregnant ♀ (n = 24 1–14 wk, n = 39 15–28 wk, n = 36 29–40 wk), 17–44 yrs 9 puerperal ♀, 19–36 yrs 7 nullipar. non-pregnant ♀, 22–33 yrs	No group difference for variation of amylase; descriptively highest values in controls; steadily decreasing values during pregnancy and lowest values puerperal.
Laine et al., 1991	Stimulated whole saliva	Basal amylase (7.30–9.30 a.m.)	11 women using OC, 24.7 ± 2.9 yrs 11 women not using OC, 29.9 ± 3.4 yrs 10 men, 31.2 ± 3.7 yrs	No effect of menstrual cycle phase; slightly higher amylase values in men.
Ciejak et al., 2007	Non-stimulated whole saliva	Basal amylase (time not specified)	64 pregnant women (21st–41st week of pregnancy), 17–39 yrs 44 non-pregnant women, 20–35 yrs	No relation between amylase activity, pregnancy and gestational age.
van Stegeren et al., 2008	Stimulated whole saliva	Basal amylase (at noon)	80 healthy adults (21 ♂, 37 OC-users, 22 non-OC), 20.7 ± 3.2 yrs	Higher overall values in men.
Diurnal profiles (more than two measurement time points)				
Rantonen and Meurman, 2000	Stimulated whole saliva	Amylase profile (8 a.m., 11 a.m., 2 p.m., 5 p.m., 8 p.m.)	30 healthy university students (14 ♀), 22.7 ± 2.8 yrs	No effect of gender, but short-term variation (independent of gender).
Nater et al., 2007	Stimulated whole saliva	Amylase profile (waking, +30 min, +60 min, every hour to 8 p.m.)	76 healthy adults (44 ♀), 18–58 yrs, 26.7 ± 8.8 yrs	No effect of gender on average amylase, men's amylase somewhat smaller linear increase and curvature over day.
Strahler et al., 2010b	Stimulated whole saliva	Amylase profile (waking, +30 min, 11 a.m., 3 p.m., 8 p.m.)	27 young dancers (15 ♀), 15–30 yrs 26 young adults(12 ♀), 20–29 yrs 31 older dancers (13 ♀), 49–75 yrs 33 older adults (14 ♀), 51–75 yrs	Effect of gender with older men lacking the typical decrease in the morning.

TSST/TSST-C, Trier Social Stress Test/Trier Social Stress Test for Children; OC, oral contraception.

2007; Granger *et al.*, 2007). Furthermore, a few studies have assessed diurnal sAA profiles and smoking and reported no or only slight changes. In summary, as a result of the toxic and thus inhibitory effects of acute tobacco consumption on sAA, and since most studies reported lower overall values in habitual smokers, smoking status is a major confounder in amylase research and studies need to be controlled for this.

Impact of alcohol

Different chemicals – including alcohol – have the potential to reflexively induce saliva secretion (Hector and Linden, 1999). In both stimulated and non-stimulated whole saliva, amylase activity was found to be decreased due to acute alcohol intake. Some human studies dealt with the question of the effects of chronic alcohol consumption on salivary gland function and revealed contradictory results showing either no differences between light drinkers and controls (Nagaya and Okuno, 1993) or decreased values in alcoholic subjects (Dutta *et al.*, 1992). In summary, evidence suggests that acute and chronic alcohol consumption is associated with dampened basal sAA activity. Until mechanisms of these functional changes are fully understood, studies should control for chronic alcohol intake and ask their participants to be abstinent before interventions and measurements.

Impact of caffeine

Caffeine can be found in many products such as tea, coffee and medications like diuretics and pain relievers. There are many reports of a specific beneficial effect of caffeine, especially in such endurance sports as cycling, running and soccer (for a review see Burke, 2008). Therefore, athletes are among those people who are interested in the effects of caffeine and researchers have to control for caffeine use. Caffeine ingestion is associated with increased sympathetic activity (Laurent *et al.*, 2000). Different studies found acute caffeine intake to be associated with higher sAA activity. However, one recent study reported no relation between habitual caffeine consumption and diurnal sAA activity (Wingenfeld *et al.*, 2010). Up to date, it is not clear whether acute stress responses of sAA differ between habitual caffeine consumers and non-consumers, and whether acute caffeine administration increases sAA activity. Studies should therefore ask their participants not to drink any coffee before experiments.

Impact of body composition

Given the fact that increases as well as decreases in body fat are accompanied by an alteration of ANS function and that body fat is a predictor of stress responsivity (Epel *et al.*, 2000; Benson *et al.*, 2009), it might be asked if body composition is a possible confounder of basal and stress-induced sAA activity. The only study investigating body fat-dependent sAA activity showed that levels were significantly higher in obese diabetic patients compared with healthy normal weight controls (Aydin, 2007). Despite the lack of studies investigating diurnal rhythmicity and sAA stress reactivity in individuals with different body compositions, it might be cautiously concluded that visceral adiposity tends to stimulate the ANS. Thus, studies investigating sAA activity should control for body fat and body composition, especially when comparing trained and untrained subjects.

Impact of food intake

Several mechanical as well as gustatory stimuli are associated with changes in salivary flow rate and composition. Both are often used to stimulate saliva flow and known to change sAA activity. To attain an ideal body composition and weight is often a central theme in different sports not only for aesthetic and performance reasons, but also according to competition specific criteria. Therefore, many athletes undergo diets while in training or preparing for an event. Investigating the effects of specific diets or dietary changes on sAA activity in normal healthy subjects revealed no differences.

An interesting study was conducted by Perry and colleagues (2007) who employed a more phylogenetic approach. The authors found that sAA gene copy numbers were positively correlated with sAA levels, which implies ethnic differences in basal and possibly stress-induced sAA activity. Taken together, there is some evidence for an association between long-term diet and sAA production. Conclusive evidence concerning the impact of gustatory and mechanical stimuli as well as real food intake on acute sAA secretion points attention to the control of time of food intake in studies measuring diurnal as well as stress-induced sAA levels. There are virtually no studies investigating the effects of dieting in athletes.

Impact of somatic and psychiatric disease

We are in the very early days of research into sport-related diseases. While there are virtually no studies conducted on this issue in athletes, experiences in other research areas could provide first insights. For instance, Bugdayci and colleagues found sAA to be related to different periods of migraine headache (Bugdayci *et al.*, 2010). Future research needs to expand to sport-related headache and trauma. Within this context, Shirasaki and colleagues (2007) reported a significant correlation between sAA levels and subjective pain intensity. Since athletes are at risk for several types of infectious disease (for a short review see Nieman, 2000), especially in competitive sports, acute infections are another issue of interest. However, so far no studies have dealt with sAA in acute infectious disease.

Competitive athletes are highly powerful but also exposed to high demands. Therefore, several psychological conditions and psychiatric disorders are common among athletes and need to be considered (for a review see Hoyer and Kleinert, 2010). However, studies investigating sAA levels in psychological disorders are rare and none have looked at athlete populations. Disorders of interest which are also present in athletes include depression and distress; anxiety-related conditions; eating disorders, especially when weight and appearance are important criteria of success such as in gymnastics or figure skating; or substance-induced disturbances. To date, only a few studies have investigated acute sAA responses in psychological disorders either in athletes or other populations (e.g. Nater and colleagues, 2010, who reported attenuated sAA responses in female patients with borderline personality disorder). In summary, somatic and psychiatric diseases have been shown to be linked to changes in amylase and because of this evidence, somatic and psychiatric diseases should be carefully controlled or excluded.

Impact of medical drugs

When dealing with medication in athletes, one has to be aware that medical drugs are usually considered doping if they are on the prohibited list of the World Anti-Doping Agency (WADA, 2011). However, among others, the use of pain-killers and anti-inflammatories is often seen in athletes. As already mentioned, sAA activity may be reduced by blockade and increased via activation of beta-adrenergic receptors (Speirs *et al.*, 1974; van Stegeren *et al.*, 2006). Thus, studies should control for substances that may change adrenergic activity, including: anti-asthmatics, anticholinergics, diuretics and antihypertensive agents, and psychopharmaceuticals (Parvinen *et al.*, 1984). Furthermore, little is known about the effect of chronic intake of adrenergically active substances on diurnal rhythms and stress responses of sAA, and studies should control for this variable.

Impact of sport on amylase (re-)activity

Impact of acute exercise

It is known that sympathetic activity increases progressively with intensity of exercise (Stainsby and Brooks, 1990) which in turn alters salivary composition (Chicharro *et al.*, 1998; Bishop *et al.*, 2000; Walsh *et al.*, 2004) including salivary alpha-amylase (Sariri and Damirchi, 2010). In studies using different kinds of physical stimulation, a sympathetic-like response was shown for salivary alpha-amylase (see Table 6.4) with rapid increases (compared with the HPA axis marker cortisol) immediately after the stressor and rapidly declining values afterwards, either in morning or afternoon exercise sessions (Li and Gleeson, 2004). Interestingly, caffeine intake prior to physical activity is able to potentiate sAA increases (Bishop *et al.*, 2006). One biological mechanism that might explain exercise-induced sAA changes is the effect of exercise-induced dehydration on saliva flow and protein content. Walsh and colleagues (2004) showed that acute dehydration led to a decrease in saliva flow. This was accompanied by increasing values of total protein concentration, while secretion rates did not change.

Impact of fitness and training status

In contrast to the multitude of studies on acute sAA responses to exercise, only little is known about the impact of fitness and training status. To the best of our knowledge there are no studies investigating whether endurance-trained individuals differ from sedentary individuals with regard to their acute, stress-induced sAA activity. However, there is evidence that sAA could serve as a non-invasive marker of aerobic fitness as it is highly positively correlated with lactate (Calvo *et al.*, 1997; Bronas *et al.*, 2002; de Oliveira *et al.*, 2010). Comparing ballroom dancers with relatively inactive controls revealed changes in diurnal sAA activity depending on age (Strahler *et al.*, 2010b). One recent study showed that low-intensity activity seems to have little relevance (Nater *et al.*, 2007), while extensive physical activity prior to testing should be avoided or controlled for.

Psychosocial stress in sport

Another issue often considered in athletes is social stress in terms of the competition aspect of many sports (for a review see Salvador and Costa, 2009). However, the majority of research relevant to this question has focused on cortisol and testosterone, rather than sAA. Only a few studies have looked at autonomic measures such as cardiovascular parameters or sAA. Kivlighan and Granger (2006) were one of the first who reported sAA responses to competition. They examined 42 members of a university rowing team and their response to a rowing ergometer competition. Alpha-amylase increased in response to the stressor in both varsity and novice athletes, with higher values for more experienced athletes across the whole competition. Furthermore, pre-competition sAA in particular was positively associated with performance.

Another sport well known for its social-evaluative and stress-inducing components is competitive ballroom dancing. However, study into possible physiological consequences in this field is only just beginning and, again, mainly focused on HPA axis activity. In 2007, Rohleder and colleagues published a paper that describes five studies designed to examine the salivary cortisol response to competitive ballroom dancing (Rohleder *et al.*, 2007). The authors began to explore this issue after having talked to amateur ballroom dancers who reported a strong subjective stress perception during competition and an increased susceptibility to disease in times of many competitions. The first study showed that competitive dancing results in strong increases of salivary cortisol compared to a control day. In contrast to the previous assumption with regard to physiological exercise-induced changes, the second study showed that dancing the same dances on a normal training day without being judged did not result in significant cortisol increases. This led the authors to conclude that ballroom dancing might serve as a paradigm for a real-life social-evaluative threat. In study three, this real-life stress response was compared with responses to a social-evaluative laboratory stressor and found to be greater. Further, cortisol stress responses were independent of experience and did not habituate across at least three competitions. The

Table 6.4 Summary of exercise and fitness effects on stress-induced and basal salivary α-amylase activity

Study	Measure/ stressor	Design	Subjects	Results
Chatterton et al., 1996	Exercise (cycling)	−45, −30, −15, −1, +1, +15, +30, +45 min	Healthy young men	3-fold increase in amylase due to aerobic exercise.
Steerenberg et al., 1997	Triathlon (stimulated whole saliva)	ø −41 min, end task	42 triathletes (6 ♀), 34.1 ± 7.3 yrs	Increase in amylase immediately after triathlon.
Calvo et al., 1997	Progressive treadmill test (non-stimulated whole saliva)	Pre, at the end of each 5 min stage	20 healthy males (military training course), 21 ± 3 yrs	Positive association amylase and lactate (amylase as non-invasive marker of aerobic fitness); increase in amylase with intense exercise.
Bishop et al., 2000	2 h cycling at 60% Vo_{2max} (non-stimulated whole saliva)	Pre, after exercising for 1 h, 2 h, 1 h postexercise	15 recreationally active men glucose (60 g/L) or placebo drink before (400 mL), during (150 mL every 15 min), and after (400 mL) the exercise or RFI with 200 mL placebo fluid during exercise), ø 20 yrs	Saliva flow rate higher on the glucose treatment compared with RFI; amylase activity and secretion rate increased due to exercise, unaffected by treatment.
Bronas et al., 2002	Incremental load Vo_2 test on a cycle ergometer	Every 3 min	9 adults, 25.3 ± 4.6 yrs	Positive association amylase and blood lactate; inversely related to heart rate.
Li and Gleeson, 2004	Cycling at 60% Vo_{2max}	−10 min, exercising for 1 h, 2 h, 1 and 2 h postexercise	8 healthy men	Amylase increase, independent of time of day; a 3 h rest enough to recover from strenuous exercise.
Kivlighan and Granger, 2006	Rowing ergometer competition	Pre, +20, +40 min	14 (4 ♀) varsity rowers, 17–31 yrs; 28 (17 ♀) novice rowers, 17–31 yrs	156% amylase increase in response to the ergometer competition; amylase higher across the competition for varsity compared to novice rowers; positive association amylase and performance and interest in team-bonding.
Bishop et al., 2006	Cycling 90 min at 70% Vo_{2max} (non-stimulated whole saliva)	−1, mid-exercise, +1, +60 min, +3.5 h	11 endurance-trained men, 23 ± 1 yrs	Increase in amylase due to caffeine intake; no return to baseline at 3.5 h post; exercise increased amylase activity and secretion, independent of caffeine intake; higher overall values in caffeine group.

Table 6.4 Continued

Study	Measure/ stressor	Design	Subjects	Results
Allgrove et al., 2008	Incremental test to exhaustion	Pre, immediately post, +1 h	10 healthy active men, ⌀ 23 yrs	No change in saliva flow rate, cycling at 75% Vo_{2max} and to exhaustion increased the secretion of amylase, independent of exercise intensity.
de Oliveira et al., 2010	Incremental effort test (50 W load, +25 W every 2 min up to exhaustion)	Pre, during exhaustion, post	12 male cyclist, 22.62 ± 3.51 yrs	Increase in amylase during the test; strong association amylase and blood lactate ($r = 0.84$).
Sariri and Damirchi, 2010	Incremental treadmill run test to exhaustion	Pre, immediately post, +1 h	12 healthy male students, 23.22 ± 2.34 yrs	At 50%, 75% Vo_{2max} and to exhaustion caused increase in amylase immediately after exercise; at 50% and 75% amylase returned to baseline, runs to exhaustion returned to about 120% baseline.
Chiodo et al., 2011	Taekwondo competition	Pre, end task, +30 min	16 young athletes (6 ♀), 13–14 yrs	115% amylase increase at the end of match, within 30 minutes of recovery return to baseline level; no gender difference.
Strahler et al., 2011	Ballroom dancing competition	Pre, end first round, +30 min, 8 p.m.	32 younger dancer (18 ♀), 21.4 ± 4.0 yrs 37 senior dancer (17 ♀), 60.6 ± 7.8 yrs	Increase in amylase after the first round; higher response in senior dancers; no association amylase response and subjective stress experiences.
Nater et al., 2007	Stimulated whole saliva	Amylase profile (waking, +30 min, +60 min, every hour to 8 p.m.)	76 healthy adults (44 ♀), 18–58 yrs, 26.7 ± 8.8 yrs	No effect of low-intensity activity on amylase.
Strahler et al., 2010b	Stimulated whole saliva	Amylase profile (waking, +30 min, 11 a.m., 3 p.m., 8 p.m.)	27 young dancers (15 ♀), 15–30 yrs 26 young adults(12♀), 20–29 yrs 31 older dancers (13 ♀), 49–75 yrs 33 older adults (14 ♀), 51–75 yrs	Flattened daily amylase slope in younger dancers and older controls; higher overall amylase output in older adults; younger male dancers and older male controls lowest amylase change after awakening.

Vo_{2max}, maximal oxygen consumption; RFI, reduced fluid intake.

last study described in this report examined the difference between dancing as a couple or dancing in a group of couples (formation dancing). Cortisol responses were mostly elevated during couple dancing, which suggests larger physiological stress responses under highly focused conditions of social-evaluative threat. Looking at the acute response of sAA to a dancing tournament, we found sAA to be increased 122% in response to the competition (Strahler *et al.*, 2011) which supports the role of ballroom dancing as being a strong real-life stressor activating the ANS.

In subsequent years, another project was designed to examine the effects of this chronic, non-habituating psychosocial stressor of competitive ballroom dancing on basal physiological functions, including sAA, this new marker of autonomic activity. We investigated the diurnal rhythmicity of salivary cortisol and alpha-amylase (Strahler *et al.*, 2010b) as well as possible effects of age and potential stress-related alterations. With respect to sAA, we found higher overall levels of sAA in both older ballroom dancers and older controls. Looking at diurnal profiles, younger male dancers showed a flattened daily variation of sAA which might be an effect of repeated stressful experiences at a younger age. Another interesting finding was a significantly negative correlation between the amount of physical activity and overall output of sAA. This might indicate a lower basal sympathetic activity in subjects who were more physically active and is therefore in line with the hypothesis of an exercise-induced attenuation of autonomic activity.

Summary and recommendations

As already noted by Goldstein (2003) ideas and research about stress must go beyond the investigation of just one effector system and just one examined variable such as the HPA axis and cortisol. Salivary alpha-amylase, therefore, has the potential to be incorporated into multisystem approaches investigating multiple homeostatic systems that are regulated in parallel. In the past two decades, knowledge about the usefulness of sAA as a marker of heightened autonomic activity has accumulated and supports this idea. Research regarding possible confounders and behavioural concomitants is also starting and provides insights into possible areas of application. Taking the next step, future studies will have to focus on the integration of sAA assessment into longitudinal studies and different research areas, including sport science, to prove its applicability as a marker of sympathetic neural functioning.

Researchers need to consider a number of variables that can influence both basal levels of sAA and acute responses of the enzyme. For the general design of studies in sport science, Table 6.5 summarizes these potential influencing factors and provides recommendations for their control.

Table 6.5 Summary of recommendations for saliva sampling and storage, and control of possible contributing factors when assessing alpha-amylase

Sampling	• Either oral swabs or passive drooling depending on practical considerations; oral swabs should be preferred in field studies (less problematic monitoring and instruction).
	• Assessing acute stress-induced changes = baseline, immediately end task, every 10 min until 20–30 min.
	• Assessing diurnal rhythm = always relative to awakening, ideally after waking up, 30 and 60 min later, and equally distributed throughout the rest of the day.
Storage	• Storing at room temperature up to 2 wks.
	• Freeze (prevent mould and bacterial growth) as soon as possible.
	• Long-term storage at –20°C or colder.
Age	• Acute stress responses are absent in newborns, can be measured in infants as young as six months, develop during childhood depending on the intervention, reach adult levels in adolescence and again attenuate in older adulthood.
	• The level of basal amylase activity changes over the lifespan.
Sex steroid influences	• Current data do not support gender differences in basal and stress-induced amylase activity as well as no effect of menstrual cycle phase.
	• Data regarding the impact of pregnancy remains inconclusive.
	• Acute amylase responses attenuated in pregnant women.
	• No systematic studies examining acute stress-induced amylase changes in different phases of the menstrual cycle.
Smoking	• Toxic and thus inhibitory effects of acute tobacco consumption on amylase.
	• Most studies reported lower overall values in habitual smokers.
	• Smoking status is a major confounder in amylase research and studies need to be controlled for this.
Alcohol	• Acute and chronic alcohol consumption associated with dampened basal amylase activity.
	• Studies should control for chronic alcohol intake and ask their participants to be abstinent before interventions and measurements.
Caffeine	• No data whether acute stress responses of amylase differ between habitual caffeine consumers and non-consumers, and whether acute caffeine administration increases amylase.
	• Studies should therefore ask their participants not to drink any coffee before experiments.
Body composition	• Especially visceral adiposity tends to stimulate the autonomic nervous system.
	• Studies investigating amylase should control for body fat and body composition.
Food intake	• First evidence for an association between long-term (evolutionary) diet and sAA production.
	• Considerable impact of gustatory and mechanical stimuli as well as real food intake on acute amylase secretion.
	• Recommended to control for time of food intake in studies measuring diurnal as well as stress- induced amylase.
Somatic and psychiatric disease	• Somatic and psychiatric diseases shown to be linked to lower and higher amylase concentrations.
	• Somatic and psychiatric diseases should therefore be carefully controlled or excluded.

Medical drugs	• Little knowledge about the chronic intake of adrenergic active substances on stress responses and diurnal rhythmicity of amylase.
	• Studies should control for substances that may change adrenergic activity including: antiasthmatics, anticholinergics, diuretics and antihypertensive agents, and psychopharmaca.
Physical activity and fitness level	• Physical activity acutely elevates amylase.
	• Hardly any data on basal or response differences between well-trained and sedentary individuals.
	• Exercise should be avoided before experiments (if not intended), physical activity of lower intensity appears to have lesser impact.

References

Adamopoulos, D., van de Borne, P. and Argacha, J. F. (2008). New insights into the sympathetic, endothelial and coronary effects of nicotine. *Clinical and Experimental Pharmacology and Physiology*, 35, 458–463.

Aguirre, A., Levine, M. J., Cohen, R. E. and Tabak, L. A. (1987). Immunochemical quantitation of alpha-amylase and secretory IgA in parotid saliva from people of various ages. *Archives of Oral Biology*, 32, 297–301.

Allgrove, J. E., Gomes, E., Hough, J. and Gleeson, M. (2008). Effects of exercise intensity on salivary antimicrobial proteins and markers of stress in active men. *Journal of Sports Sciences*, 26, 653–661.

Anderson, L. C., Garrett, J. R., Johnson, D. A., Kauffman, D. L., Keller, P. J. and Thulin, A. (1984). Influence of circulating catecholamines on protein secretion into rat parotid saliva during parasympathetic stimulation. *Journal of Physiology*, 352, 163–171.

Artino, M., Dragomir, M., Ionescu, S., Bădia, D., Niţă, V. and Chiţoi, E. (1998). Diurnal behaviour of some salivary parameters in patients with diabetes mellitus (protein concentration, amylase activity, density) – note I. Romanian *Journal of Physiology*, 35, 79–84.

Aydin, S. (2007). A comparison of ghrelin, glucose, alpha-amylase and protein levels in saliva from diabetics. *Journal of Biochemistry and Molecular Biology*, 40, 29–35.

Beltzer, E. K., Fortunato, C. K., Guaderrama, M. M., *et al.* (2010). Salivary flow and alpha-amylase: collection technique, duration, and oral fluid type. *Physiology and Behavior*, 101, 289–296.

Ben-Aryeh, H., Fisher, M., Szargel, R. and Laufer, D. (1990). Composition of whole unstimulated saliva of healthy children: changes with age. *Archives of Oral Biology*, 35, 929–931.

Benson, S., Arck, P. C., Tan, S., *et al.* (2009). Effects of obesity on neuroendocrine, cardiovascular, and immune cell responses to acute psychosocial stress in premenopausal women. *Psychoneuroendocrinology*, 34, 181–189.

Bhoola, K. D., Matthews, R. W. and Roberts, F. (1978). A survey of salivary kallikrein and amylase in a population of schoolgirls, throughout the menstrual cycle. *Clinical Science and Molecular Medicine – Supplement*, 55, 561–566.

Bishop, N. C., Blannin, A. K., Armstrong, E., Rickman, M. and Gleeson, M. (2000). Carbohydrate and fluid intake affect the saliva flow rate and IgA response to cycling. *Medicine and Science in Sports and Exercise*, 32, 2046–2051.

Bishop, N. C., Walker, G. J., Scanlon, G. A., Richards, S. and Rogers, E. (2006). Salivary IgA responses to prolonged intensive exercise following caffeine ingestion. *Medicine and Science in Sports and Exercise*, 38, 513–519.

Bronas, U., Sukalski, K., Brinkert, R. and von Duvillard, S. P. (2002). Determination of the anaerobic threshold by analysis of salivary alpha-amylase and blood lactate. *Medicine and Science in Sports and Exercise*, 34, S150.

Bugdayci, G., Yildiz, S., Altunrende, B., Yildiz, N. and Alkoy, S. (2010). Salivary alpha amylase activity in migraine patients. *Autonomic Neuroscience*, 155, 121–124.

Burke, L. M. (2008). Caffeine and sports performance. *Applied Physiology, Nutrition, and Metabolism*, 33, 1319–1334.

Calvo, F., Chicharro, J. L., Bandres, F., *et al.* (1997). Anaerobic threshold determination with analysis of salivary amylase. *Canadian Journal of Applied Physiology*, 22, 553–561.

Chatterton, R. T., Jr., Vogelsong, K. M., Lu, Y. C., Ellman, A. B. and Hudgens, G. A. (1996). Salivary alpha-amylase as a measure of endogenous adrenergic activity. *Clinical Physiology*, 16, 433–448.

Chicharro, J. L., Lucia, A., Perez, M., Vaquero, A. F. and Urena, R. (1998). Saliva composition and exercise. *Sports Medicine*, 26, 17–27.

Chiodo, S., Tessitore, A., Cortis, C., *et al.* (2011). Stress-related hormonal and psychological changes to official youth Taekwondo competitions. *Scandinavian Journal of Medicine and Science in Sports*, 21, 111–119.

Ciejak, M., Olszewska, M., Jakubowska, K., Zebielowicz, D., Safranow, K. and Chlubek, D. (2007). Activity of alpha-amylase and concentration of protein in saliva of pregnant women. *Annales Academiae Medicae Stetinensis*, 53, 42–45.

D'Alessandro, S., Curbelo, H. M., Tumilasci, O. R., Tessler, J. A. and Houssay, A. B. (1989). Changes in human parotid salivary protein and sialic acid levels during pregnancy. *Archives of Oral Biology*, 34, 829–831.

Davis, E. P. and Granger, D. A. (2009). Developmental differences in infant salivary alpha-amylase and cortisol responses to stress. *Psychoneuroendocrinology*, 34, 795–804.

Dawes, C. (1972). Circadian rhythms in human salivary flow rate and composition. *Journal of Physiology*, 220, 529–545.

de Oliveira, V. N., Bessa, A., Lamounier, R. P., de Santana, M. G., de Mello, M. T. and Espindola, F. S. (2010). Changes in the salivary biomarkers induced by an effort test. *International Journal of Sports Medicine*, 31, 377–381.

DeCaro, J. A. (2008). Methodological considerations in the use of salivary alpha-amylase as a stress marker in field research. *American Journal of Human Biology*, 20, 617–619.

Dutta, S. K., Orestes, M., Vengulekur, S. and Kwo, P. (1992). Ethanol and human saliva: effect of chronic alcoholism on flow rate, composition, and epidermal growth factor. *American Journal of Gastroenterology*, 87, 350–354.

Ehlert, U., Erni, K., Hebisch, G. and Nater, U. (2006). Salivary alpha-amylase levels after yohimbine challenge in healthy men. *Journal of Clinical Endocrinology and Metabolism*, 91, 5130–5133.

Epel, E. S., McEwen, B., Seeman, T., *et al.* (2000). Stress and body shape: stress-induced cortisol secretion is consistently greater among women with central fat. *Psychosomatic Medicine*, 62, 623–632.

Ferguson, D. B., Fort, A., Elliott, A. L. and Potts, A. J. (1973). Circadian rhythms in human parotid saliva flow rate and composition. *Archives of Oral Biology*, 18, 1155–1173.

Froehlich, D. A., Pangborn, R. M. and Whitaker, J. R. (1987). The effect of oral stimulation on human parotid salivary flow rate and alpha-amylase secretion. *Physiology and Behavior*, 41, 209–217.

Garrett, J. R. (1987). The proper role of nerves in salivary secretion: a review. *Journal of Dental Research*, 66, 387–397.

Gasteiger, E., Hoogland, C., Gattiker, A., *et al.* (2005). Protein identification and analysis tools on the ExPASy server. In J. M. Walker (ed.), *The Proteomics Protocols Handbook* (pp. 571–607). Totowa: Humana Press.

Goi, N., Hirai, Y., Harada, H., *et al.* (2007). Comparison of peroxidase response to mental arithmetic stress in saliva of smokers and non-smokers. *Journal of Toxicological Sciences*, 32, 121–127.

Goldstein, D. S. (2003). Catecholamines and stress. *Endocrine Regulations*, 37, 69–80.

Gordis, E. B., Granger, D. A., Susman, E. J. and Trickett, P. K. (2008). Salivary alpha amylase-cortisol asymmetry in maltreated youth. *Hormones and Behavior*, 53, 96–103.

Granger, D. A., Blair, C., Willoughby, M., *et al.* (2007). Individual differences in salivary cortisol and alpha-amylase in mothers and their infants: relation to tobacco smoke exposure. *Developmental Psychobiology*, 49, 692–701.

Groer, M., Murphy, R., Bunnell, W., *et al.* (2010). Salivary measures of stress and immunity in police officers engaged in simulated critical incident scenarios. *Journal of Occupational and Environmental Medicine*, 52, 595–602.

Hector, M. P. and Linden, R. W. (1999). Reflexes of salivary secretion. In J. R. Garrett, J. Ekstrom and L. C. Anderson (eds), *Neural Mechanisms of Salivary Gland Secretion. Frontiers in Oral Biology*, Volume 11 (pp. 196–218). Basel: Karger.

Hodge, C., Lebenthal, E., Lee, P. C. and Topper, W. (1983). Amylase in the saliva and in the gastric aspirates of premature infants: its potential role in glucose polymer hydrolysis. *Pediatric Research*, 17, 998–1001.

Hoyer, J. and Kleinert, J. (2010). Leistungssport und psychische störungen. *Psychotherapeutenjournal*, 9, 252–260.

Jenzano, J. W., Brown, C. K. and Mauriello, S. M. (1987). Temporal variation of glandular kallikrein, protein and amylase in mixed human saliva. *Archives of Oral Biology*, 32, 757–759.

Kang, Y. (2010). Psychological stress-induced changes in salivary alpha-amylase and adrenergic activity. *Nursing and Health Science*, 12, 477–484.

Kirschbaum, C. and Hellhammer, D. H. (1999). Hypothalamus-hypophysen-nebennierenrindenachse. In D. H. Hellhammer and C. Kirschbaum (eds), *Enzyklopädie der Psychologie. Psychoendokrinologie und Psychoimmunologie, Biologische Psychologie*, Volume 3 (pp. 79–140). Göttingen: Hogrefe.

Kirschbaum, C., Kudielka, B. M., Gaab, J., Schommer, N. C. and Hellhammer, D. H. (1999). Impact of gender, menstrual cycle phase, and oral contraceptives on the activity of the hypothalamus-pituitary-adrenal axis. *Psychosomatic Medicine*, 61, 154–162.

Kivlighan, K. T. and Granger, D. A. (2006). Salivary alpha-amylase response to competition: relation to gender, previous experience, and attitudes. *Psychoneuroendocrinology*, 31, 703–714.

Laine, M., Pienihakkinen, K., Ojanotko-Harri, A. and Tenovuo, J. (1991). Effects of low-dose oral contraceptives on female whole saliva. *Archives of Oral Biology*, 36, 549–552.

Laurent, D., Schneider, K. E., Prusaczyk, W. K., *et al.* (2000). Effects of caffeine on muscle glycogen utilization and the neuroendocrine axis during exercise. *Journal of Clinical Endocrinology and Metabolism*, 85, 2170–2175.

Li, T. L. and Gleeson, M. (2004). The effect of single and repeated bouts of prolonged cycling and circadian variation on saliva flow rate, immunoglobulin A and alpha-amylase responses. *Journal of Sports Sciences*, 22, 1015–1024.

Mackie, D. A. and Pangborn, R. M. (1990). Mastication and its influence on human salivary flow and alpha-amylase secretion. *Physiology and Behavior*, 47, 593–595.

Maldonado, E. F., Fernandez, F. J., Trianes, M. V., *et al.* (2008). Cognitive performance and morning levels of salivary cortisol and alpha-amylase in children reporting high vs. low daily stress perception. *Spanish Journal of Psychology*, 11, 3–15.

McKay, K. A., Buen, J. E., Bohan, K. J. and Maye, J. P. (2010). Determining the relationship of acute stress, anxiety and salivary alpha-amylase level with performance of student nurse anesthetists during human-based anesthesia simulator training. *AANA (American Association of Nurse Anesthetists) Journal*, 78, 301–309.

Michaud, D. S., Miller, S. M., Ferrarotto, C., Konkle, A. T., Keith, S. E. and Campbell, K. B. (2006). Waking levels of salivary biomarkers are altered following sleep in a lab with no further increase associated with simulated night-time noise exposure. *Noise Health*, 8, 30–39.

Nagaya, T. and Okuno, M. (1993). No effects of smoking or drinking habits on salivary amylase. *Toxicology Letters*, 66, 257–261.

Nater, U. M., Rohleder, N., Gaab, J., *et al.* (2005). Human salivary alpha-amylase reactivity in a psychosocial stress paradigm. *International Journal of Psychophysiology*, 55, 333–342.

Nater, U. M., La Marca, R., Florin, L., *et al.* (2006). Stress-induced changes in human salivary alpha-amylase activity – associations with adrenergic activity. *Psychoneuroendocrinology*, 31, 49–58.

Nater, U. M., Rohleder, N., Schlotz, W., Ehlert, U. and Kirschbaum, C. (2007). Determinants of the diurnal course of salivary alpha-amylase. *Psychoneuroendocrinology*, 32, 392–401.

Nater, U. M., Bohus, M., Abbruzzese, E., *et al.* (2010). Increased psychological and attenuated cortisol and alpha-amylase responses to acute psychosocial stress in female patients with borderline personality disorder. *Psychoneuroendocrinology*, 35, 1565–1572.

Nieman, D. C. (2000). Exercise, the immune system, and infectious disease. In W. E. G. Jr and D.T.Kirkendall (eds), *Exercise and Sport Science* (pp. 177–190). Philadelphia: Lippincott Williams and Wilkins.

Nierop, A., Bratsikas, A., Klinkenberg, A., Nater, U. M., Zimmermann, R. and Ehlert, U. (2006). Prolonged salivary cortisol recovery in second-trimester pregnant women and attenuated salivary alpha-amylase responses to psychosocial stress in human pregnancy. *Journal of Clinical Endocrinology and Metabolism*, 91, 1329–1335.

O'Donnell, K., Kammerer, M., O'Reilly, R., Taylor, A. and Glover, V. (2009). Salivary alpha-amylase stability, diurnal profile and lack of response to the cold hand test in young women. *Stress*, 12, 549–554.

Parvinen, T., Parvinen, I. and Larmas, M. (1984). Stimulated salivary flow rate, pH and lactobacillus and yeast concentrations in medicated persons. *Scandinavian Journal of Dental Research*, 92, 524–532.

Perroni, F., Tessitore, A., Cibelli, G., *et al.* (2009). Effects of simulated firefighting on the responses of salivary cortisol, alpha-amylase and psychological variables. *Ergonomics*, 52, 484–491.

Perry, G. H., Dominy, N. J., Claw, K. G., *et al.* (2007). Diet and the evolution of human amylase gene copy number variation. *Nature Genetics*, 39, 1256–1260.

Pilardeau, P., Richalet, J. P., Bouissou, P., Vaysse, J., Larmignat, P. and Boom, A. (1990). Saliva flow and composition in humans exposed to acute altitude hypoxia. *European Journal of Applied Physiology and Occupational Physiology*, 59, 450–453.

Pruessner, J. C., Kirschbaum, C., Meinlschmid, G. and Hellhammer, D. H. (2003). Two formulas for computation of the area under the curve represent measures of total hormone concentration versus time-dependent change. *Psychoneuroendocrinology*, 28, 916–931.

Rai, B. and Kaur, J. (2011). Salivary stress markers and psychological stress in simulated microgravity: 21 days in 6 degrees head-down tilt. *Journal of Oral Science*, 53, 103–107.

Rantonen, P. J. and Meurman, J. H. (2000). Correlations between total protein, lysozyme, immunoglobulins, amylase, and albumin in stimulated whole saliva during daytime. *Acta Odontologica Scandinavica*, 58, 160–165.

Rohleder, N. and Nater, U. M. (2009). Determinants of salivary alpha-amylase in humans and methodological considerations. *Psychoneuroendocrinology*, 34, 469–485.

Rohleder, N., Nater, U. M., Wolf, J. M., Ehlert, U. and Kirschbaum, C. (2004). Psychosocial stress-induced activation of salivary alpha-amylase: an indicator of sympathetic activity? *Annals of the New York Academy of Sciences*, 1032, 258–263.

Rohleder, N., Wolf, J. M., Maldonado, E. F. and Kirschbaum, C. (2006). The psychosocial stress-induced increase in salivary alpha-amylase is independent of saliva flow rate. *Psychophysiology*, 43, 645–652.

Rohleder, N., Beulen, S. E., Chen, E., Wolf, J. M. and Kirschbaum, C. (2007). Stress on the dance floor: the cortisol stress response to social-evaluative threat in competitive ballroom dancers. *Personality and Social Psychology Bulletin*, 33, 69–84.

Rohleder, N., Chen, E., Wolf, J. M. and Miller, G. E. (2008). The psychobiology of trait shame in young women: extending the social self preservation theory. *Health Psychology*, 27, 523–532.

Salvador, A. and Costa, R. (2009). Coping with competition: neuroendocrine responses and cognitive variables. *Neuroscience and Biobehavioral Reviews*, 33, 160–170.

Sariri, R. and Damirchi, A. (2010). Alternation in salivary alpha-amylase due to exercise intensity. *Pharmacologyonline*, 3, 263–269.

Schaffer, L., Burkhardt, T., Muller-Vizentini, D., *et al.* (2008). Cardiac autonomic balance in small-for-gestational-age neonates. *American Journal of Physiology – Heart and Circulatory Physiology*, 294, H884–890.

Schoofs, D., Hartmann, R. and Wolf, O. T. (2008). Neuroendocrine stress responses to an oral academic examination: no strong influence of sex, repeated participation and personality traits. *Stress*, 11, 52–61.

Sevenhuysen, G. P., Holodinsky, C. and Dawes, C. (1984). Development of salivary alpha-amylase in infants from birth to 5 months. *American Journal of Clinical Nutrition*, 39, 584–588.

Shirasaki, S., Fujii, H., Takahashi, M., *et al.* (2007). Correlation between salivary alpha-amylase activity and pain scale in patients with chronic pain. Regional *Anesthesia and Pain Medicine*, 32, 120–123.

Speirs, R. L., Herring, J., Cooper, W. D., Hardy, C. C. and Hind, C. R. (1974). The influence of sympathetic activity and isoprenaline on the secretion of amylase from the human parotid gland. *Archives of Oral Biology*, 19, 747–752.

Spinrad, T. L., Eisenberg, N., Granger, D. A., *et al.* (2009). Individual differences in preschoolers' salivary cortisol and alpha-amylase reactivity: relations to temperament and maladjustment. *Hormones and Behavior*, 56, 133–139.

Stainsby, W. N. and Brooks, G. A. (1990). Control of lactic acid metabolism in contracting muscles and during exercise. *Exercise and Sport Sciences Reviews*, 18, 29–63.

Steerenberg, P. A., van Asperen, I. A., van Nieuw Amerongen, A., Biewenga, A., Mol, D. and Medema, G. J. (1997). Salivary levels of immunoglobulin A in triathletes. *European Journal of Oral Sciences*, 105, 305–309.

Strahler, J., Mueller, A., Rosenloecher, F., Kirschbaum, C. and Rohleder, N. (2010a). Salivary alpha-amylase stress reactivity across different age groups. *Psychophysiology*, 47, 587–595.

Strahler, J., Berndt, C., Kirschbaum, C. and Rohleder, N. (2010b). Aging diurnal rhythms and chronic stress: Distinct alteration of diurnal rhythmicity of salivary alpha-amylase and cortisol. *Biological Psychology*, 84, 248–256.

Strahler, J., Kirschbaum, C. and Rohleder, N. (2011). Turniertanzen: Dissoziation der psychischen und physiologischen Stressreaktion. In J. Ohlert and J. Kleinert (eds), *Sport vereinT – Psychologie und Bewegung in Gesellschaft Abstractband zur 43. Jahrestagung der asp vom 2.-4. Juni 2011 in Köln* (Volume 210, Schriften der Deutschen Vereinigung für Sportwissenschaft, pp. 138). Hamburg: Edition Czwalina Feldhaus Verlag.

van Stegeren, A., Rohleder, N., Everaerd, W. and Wolf, O. T. (2006). Salivary alpha amylase as marker for adrenergic activity during stress: effect of betablockade. *Psychoneuroendocrinology*, 31, 137–141.

van Stegeren, A., Wolf, O. T. and Kindt, M. (2008). Salivary alpha amylase and cortisol responses to different stress tasks: impact of sex. *International Journal of Psychophysiology*, 69, 33–40.

WADA (2011). The World Anti-Doping Code The 2011 Prohibited List International Standard. Retrieved from http://www.wada-ama.org (retrieved 12 June 2011).

Walsh, N. P., Montague, J. C., Callow, N. and Rowlands, A. V. (2004). Saliva flow rate, total protein concentration and osmolality as potential markers of whole body hydration status during progressive acute dehydration in humans. *Archives of Oral Biology*, 49, 149–154.

Wingenfeld, K., Schulz, M., Damkroeger, A., Philippsen, C., Rose, M. and Driessen, M. (2010). The diurnal course of salivary alpha-amylase in nurses: an investigation of potential confounders and associations with stress. *Biological Psychology*, 85, 179–181.

Witt, R. L. (2006). *Salivary Gland Diseases: Surgical and Medical Management*. Stuttgart: Thieme.

Wolf, J. M., Nicholls, E. and Chen, E. (2008). Chronic stress, salivary cortisol, and alpha-amylase in children with asthma and healthy children. *Biological Psychology*, 78, 20–28.

Yamaguchi, M., Deguchi, M. and Miyazaki, Y. (2006). The effects of exercise in forest and urban environments on sympathetic nervous activity of normal young adults. *Journal of International Medical Research*, 34, 152–159.

Part III

Research trends

Katharina Strahler and Felix Ehrlenspiel

Having described the most frequently investigated psychoneuroendocrinological parameters in the previous section, this section presents current studies investigating hormonal responses in sport and exercise. The chapters are far from comprehensive and there are many further intriguing research programmes contributing to a psychoneuroendocrinology of sport and exercise, such as the hormonal differences between home matches and away matches (e.g. Carré *et al.*, 2006; Neave and Wolfson, 2006) or the hormonal response to winning and losing (e.g. Oliveira *et al.*, 2009). However, this section provides a first insight into current themes that are of interest when doing psychoneuroendocrinological research in sport and exercise psychology. Although at first the selection appears arbitrary, each chapter represents a unique field of study in sport psychology to which a psychoneuroendocrinology of sport and exercise can contribute an understanding of physiological mechanisms.

First, Edith Filaire illustrates one of the core themes in sport psychology but also of biopsychological research on hormones in sport and exercise – competitive anxiety and the hormonal reaction in relation to sport competitions. Here, the influence of endocrinological responses on competitive anxiety and vice versa are of actual interest to sport psychologists, trainers and athletes. The chapter also suggests how psychoneuroendocrinology might add to our understanding of a 'psychology perspective' within the cognitive behavioural orientation in sport psychology. In Chapter 8, Ulrike Rimmele presents a research programme that investigates how physical fitness modulates hormonal and psychological responses to stress. Thus it represents the 'sport perspective' within the cognitive behavioural orientation in sport psychology and shows how psychoneuroendocrinology might explain the effects of sport on the mind. In Chapter 9, Silvan Steiner turns the viewpoint away from the athletes themselves and looks at spectators and their hormonal responses during sport events. Giving insights into physiological effects while watching a soccer game, the chapter discusses how psychoneuroendocrinology might add to the integration of the physiological with the social cognitive orientation in sport psychology. In the final chapter, Ferran Suay discusses the overtraining syndrome, representing the demand for integration of psychology and physiology not only from a theoretical perspective but from sheer practical needs. When athletes find themselves 'in a hole' with increasing levels of training sessions and strict competition schedules but declining performance it is the combination or rather integration of endocrinological and psychological markers that will eventually indicate and prevent negative health consequences.

References

Carré, J., Muir, C., Belanger, J. and Putnam, S. K. (2006). Pre-competition hormonal and psychological levels of elite hockey players: relationship to the 'home advantage.' *Physiology and Behavior*, 89, 392–398.

Neave, N. and Wolfson, S. (2006). Testosterone, territoriality and the 'home advantage.' *Physiology and Behavior*, 78, 269–275.

Oliveira, T., Gouveia, M. J. and Oliveira, R. F. (2009). Testosterone responsiveness to winning and losing experiences in female soccer players. *Psychoneuroendocrinology*, 34, 1056–1064.

7   The psychoneuroendocrine response to sports competition

Edith Filaire

Stress is an inherent aspect of sports competition. However, individuals perceive competition differently, with some responding positively to the challenge while others feel debilitated and performance suffers. The relationship between anxiety and sport performance has attracted much attention from researchers over the last 25 years, and to better understand the relationship between stress and performance in sport, the psychological, physiological, and less frequently, biochemical responses have been investigated. Since anxiety is a negative emotional state, characterized by nervousness, worry and apprehension and is associated with activation or arousal of the body, some studies have tended to focus on the potentially negative effects on performance. However, some authors (Jones and Swain, 1992; Woodman and Hardy, 2001) have reported that anxiety can have positive consequences in performance environments. For Cheng *et al.* (2009), the adaptive nature of anxiety may have been under-represented by the conventional two components of worry and emotionality, and they proposed a more balanced viewpoint to reflect not just the maladaptive but also adaptive aspects of anxiety.

Concomitant psychological and physiological measures are advocated in competitive stress research (Hatfield and Landers, 1983) as a broader approach to measure self-reported anxiety alone. The physiological response to stress is more recently conceptualized as an individual's psychological and physiological autonomic system activation, varying on a continuum from deep sleep to extreme excitement (Gould and Krane, 1992). Heart rate, respiration, blood pressure, skin responses, muscle tension, brain activity and neuroendocrine measures are physiological parameters evaluating the arousal state (McKay *et al.*, 1997). This chapter provides a review of the models of competitive anxiety and the neuroendocrine response to stress is also discussed. The aim of this part of the discussion is to show that adopting psychophysiological approaches, which are minimally invasive to the sportsperson, will ensure that the physiological stress responses can be measured more frequently and therefore in close proximity to performance.

Models of competitive anxiety

Before embarking on a discussion of the role of anxiety in social psychological research applied to sport performance, a prerequisite step is to define the terms anxiety and stress. The study of competitive stress and anxiety in sport has been hindered by a lack of consistency in the use of key terms (Jones *et al.*, 1993; Hardy *et al.*, 1996; Gould *et al.*, 2002). Stress has often been used interchangeably to describe a stimulus or a response of a person–environment interaction. This is the case, despite there being a clear conceptual distinction between the terms stressor and strain. *Stressors* refer to events, situations or conditions, while *strain* describes an individual's negative response to stressors.

In recent years stress research has incorporated new important concepts with strong repercussions at the conceptual and methodological levels. *Allostasis*, defined as the adaptive process for actively maintaining stability through change (Sterling and Eyer, 1988), is a fundamental process through which organisms actively adjust to both predictable and unpredictable events. It is complemented with other concepts, such as the 'allostatic load', which can be described as the cumulative impairment ('wear and tear') derived from the frequent or inefficiently managed activation of the mediators of the allostasis (hormones, neurotransmitters, cytokines, etc.; McEwen, 1998). Contemporary conceptualizations view stress not as a factor that resides in either an individual or the environment, but rather as a relationship between the two (Lazarus, 1981). Stress is regarded as a relational concept. Rather than being defined as a specific kind of external stimulation nor a specific pattern of physiological, behavioural or subjective reactions, it is viewed as a relationship (transaction) between individuals and their environment.

Lazarus and Folkman (1986) proposed two processes as central mediators within the person–environment transaction: cognitive *appraisal* and *coping* (i.e. individuals' efforts in thought and action to manage specific demands). The concept of appraisal (primary and secondary appraisal) is based on the idea that emotional processes (including stress) are dependent on actual expectancies that persons manifest with regard to the significance and outcome of a specific encounter. The situation the individual is faced with is evaluated based on the expectancies attached to it and to the possible actions available to this particular individual. Consequently, to a large degree, stress response depends on previous experience and how it is interpreted. If it is appraised by the individual as threatening to his or her physiological or psychological balance, a measurable physiological response will be produced (McEwen *et al.*, 1993).

Mason emphasized that the perception of the situation is the main factor in the neuroendocrine variability and activation (Mason *et al.*, 1973). A key concept has also been the control and, more specifically, the perceived control, that has emerged as a powerful explanatory variable in stress research.

Concerning the competitive stress in sport, Melallieu *et al.* (2009) reported that competitive stress involves a transaction between an individual and the environmental demands associated primarily and directly with competitive performance. It also includes environmental demands in relation to competitive performance (competitive stressors) and a specific negative emotional response to competitive stressors, called *competitive anxiety*. Anxiety is a specific emotion that has been described as an unpleasant feeling of apprehension and distress, and is usually accompanied by unpleasant physiological responses (Martens et al., 1990).

More than any other single emotion, anxiety has been the focus of the vast majority of research on emotion and social cognition in sport performance (Gould and Krane, 1992). Modern theorists make the distinction between *state* and *trait* anxiety. Anxiety can be both a tendency to respond with anxious symptoms in situations evaluated as being competitive and a psychological state determined by environmental factors such as competition, as well as intrapersonal variables such as the appraisal of the event as being important. Theorists also make the distinction between *arousal* and *anxiety*.

Anxiety is classed as having a *somatic* and a *cognitive* component. Somatic anxiety is conceived of as the perception of the physiological–affective elements of the anxiety experience, indications of autonomic arousal and unpleasant feeling states, such as nervousness and tension (cf. Morris and Liebert, 1973). The cognitive component is composed of cognitive elements of anxiety, such as negative expectations and cognitive concerns about oneself, the situation at hand and potential consequences (cf. Martens et al., 1990).

Arousal is a blend of physiological and psychological activity in a person, and it refers to the intensity dimensions of motivation at a particular moment. The intensity of arousal falls along a continuum ranging from not at all aroused to completely aroused (Gould and Krane, 1992). Recent appraisal theorists believe that arousal is implicated in emotional responses such as anxiety, but there are specific patterns of emotional responses according to the way in which the arousal situation is appraised.

Sport psychologists have studied the relationship between anxiety and performance for decades. Early theories proposed a simple linear relationship between arousal and performance. However, observations that very low or very high levels of arousal resulted in inferior performance of fine motor skills and complex cognitive tasks when compared to intermediate arousal levels in competitive sport led to several researchers proposing that an optimal level of arousal was the most effective for performance (Landers, 1980). This relationship was referred to as optimal arousal theory or the inverted-U hypothesis. While this theory was attractive because of its neat and clear set of predictions, it has been criticized because of its over-simplification of the role of arousal and the nature of skills within a variety of different sports (Jones, 1991).

Multidimensional anxiety theory has attempted to provide a better explanation of the relationships between anxiety and arousal by incorporating somatic anxiety as a measure of the felt symptoms of heightened arousal (Martens et al., 1990; Smith et al., 2006). In this multidimensional anxiety theory, cognitive anxiety is hypothesized as having a negative linear relationship with performance, somatic anxiety is hypothesized as having a quadratic (inverted-U shaped) relationship with performance; and self-confidence is hypothesized as having a positive linear relationship with performance.

Following a series of competitive anxiety investigations, the traditional view that increases in competitive anxiety were negative to performance was questioned, and a recent branch of research has examined the potential of heightened cognitive and somatic anxiety to have positive or facilitative effects on performance and has introduced the notion of direction into the competitive anxiety literature (Jones, 1991). Direction is defined as the interpretation of the symptoms associated with competitive anxiety as being facilitative or debilitative towards performance (Jones and Hanton, 2001). Frequency was also added and can be defined as the amount of time spent on attending to symptoms experienced concerning competition (Swain and Jones, 1993). These authors basically contended that viewing anxiety as facilitative leads to superior performance whereas viewing it as debilitative leads to poor performance. Moreover, whether the resulting state anxiety is perceived as facilitative or debilitative depends on how much control the athlete perceives they have.

Jones *et al.* (1993) proposed that the appraisal of the competitive situation as threatening as well as a secondary appraisal of coping ability, or control over resources to cope with the threatening situation, would determine whether the anxiety response would be interpreted as facilitative or debilitative. Subsequent research has also focused on the effects of competence-related variables such as ability, goal attainment and self-confidence on the relationship between the directional component of anxiety and performance. However, researchers have questioned the concept of the directional measure, that it may instead be a measure of positive affect or excitement that has been noted by Jones (1995). One additional limitation that has been levelled at Jones' (1995) control theory of facilitative–debilitative anxiety is that it does not explicitly account for the level of arousal experienced by an individual.

Edward and Hardy (1996) suggested that the relationship between anxiety intensity, direction, and performance was more complex, and reported that physiological arousal needs to be implicated in any complete model of the anxiety process in sport performance.

In line with this suggestion, Hardy (1996) adopted the catastrophe model, which predicts that physiological arousal is related to performance in an inverted-U fashion, but only when an athlete is not worried or has low cognitive state anxiety. Even if this theory is an important addition to the literature, tests of the model have been limited. Moreover, Woodman and Hardy (2001) suggested that the catastrophe approach is a model and not a theory, and therefore cannot explain the mechanisms through which the anxiety components may interact to effect performance.

An alternative approach to the study of emotion in sport performance was the Individualized Zones of Optimal Functioning (IZOF) model (Hanin, 1995). This model offers an integrative perspective on emotional experience and sport performance that adopts hypotheses from person–environment interaction theory, appraisal theories of emotion, trait–state distinctions, idiographic versus nomothetic views of personality, and psychological readiness for competition. The key principle of the IZOF model is that every athlete has an optimal level of range of emotional intensity, such as anxiety, that will lead to successful performance in sport. Hanin (2007) expanded the IZOF notion beyond anxiety to show how zones of optimal functioning use a variety of emotions and other biopsychoso-cial states, such as determination, pleasantness and laziness. The IZOF view also contends that there are positive and negative emotions that enhance perform-ance and positive and negative emotions that have a dysfunctional influence on performance. However, the theoretical underpinning of the IZOF model is questionable because it does not explain the antecedents of predictors of optimal anxiety, but instead focuses on the individual nature of the anxiety–performance relationship.

Understanding of anxiety and emotion in sport performance has been fur-thered through advancement of other models, such as Reversal Theory (Apter, 1982). This theory provides a general framework for the understanding of the relationship between arousal and emotion, and how these influence motivational constructs and behaviour. Reversal theory predicts that an individual's meta-motivational state will determine the relationship between their hedonic tone and arousal level. A metamotivational state is a person's interpretation of their motives or goals in a given context and at a given point in time. An individual can either be goal-focused or serious in their pursuit of their outcomes, known as a *telic metamotivational state*, or be activity-oriented in their approach, known as the *paratelic metamotivational state*. In a telic state, high physiological arousal will be interpreted as anxiety; whereas in a paratelic state, high physiological arousal will be experienced as excitement. Equilibrium in the desired meta-motivational state is achieved when minimal differences arise between an individual's preferred and actual arousal state. In addition, contingent upon the perceived pleasure or hedonic tone of the individual, performers can also suddenly reverse from the experience of high arousal as excitement to one of anxiety (Kerr, 1997). Unlike the inverted-U hypothesis, high levels of physiological or felt arousal may not automatically lead to detrimental performance consequences and may actually be beneficial. However, few tests of the theory's predictions have been made, so firm conclusions about the scientific predictions cannot be made. Moreover, the approach has been suggested as offering little in terms of explaining how and why anxiety (through changes in arousal states) might affect motor performance.

Recently, Fletcher and Fletcher (2005) proposed a meta-model of stress, emo-tion and performance. This model divides the stress process into three stages: (1) the person–environment fit; (2) the emotion–performance fit; and (3) the subsequent coping and overall outcome. The negative consequence of any incon-gruence in the first stage represents the competitive anxiety response (i.e. psy-chological strain associated with a negative primary and secondary appraisal of a competitive stressor). Similar to the model of control proposed by Jones (1995), whereby individual differences were hypothesized to influence symptom inter-pretation, this meta-model also predicts that the competitive stress process is moderated by various personal and situational characteristics, such as individual differences, trait anxiety, cognitive bias, positive and negative affect, self-confi-dence, neuroticism and extraversion, hardiness, coping strategies, psychological study, gender, skill and performance level, control, and achievement motivation (Melallieu *et al.*, 2009).

More recently, Jones *et al.* (2009) proposed a Theory of Challenge and Threat States in Athletes (TCTSA), which is an amalgamation and extension of the biopsychosocial model of challenge and threat, the model of adaptive approaches to competition and the debilitative and facilitative competitive state anxiety model. In the TCTSA, the researchers posit that self-efficacy, perceptions of control and achievement goals determine challenge or threat states in response to competition. Distinct patterns of neuroendocrine and cardiovascular responses are indicative of a challenge or threat state. Increases in adrenaline and cardiac activity and a decrease in total peripheral vascular resistance (TPR) characterize a challenge state and increases in cortisol, smaller increases in cardiac activity and either no change or an increase in TPR characterize a threat state. Positive and negative emotions can occur in a challenge state while a threat state is associated with negative emotions only. Emotions are perceived as helpful to performance in a challenge state but not in a threat state. Challenge and threat states influence effort, attention, decision-making and physical functioning, and accordingly, sport performance.

Finally, an integrated three-dimensional model of performance anxiety was constructed to offer an alternative conceptualization that may contribute to understanding of the complex anxiety–performance relationship (Cheng *et al.*, 2009). In particular, the adaptive potential (producing positive effects) of anxiety was acknowledged explicitly by including a regulatory dimension. This model is characterized by five subcomponents, with worry and self-focused attention representing cognitive anxiety, autonomous hyperactivity and somatic tension representing physiological anxiety, and perceived control representing the regulatory dimension of anxiety. Preliminary research has supported the application of this three-dimensional conceptualization of performance anxiety in Taekwondo (Cheng *et al.*, 2011).

Neuroendocrine studies of competitive anxiety

The neuroendocrine response (i.e. the release of hormones) as part of the physiological stress response has seen a surge in interest in recent years concerning anxiety and stress research in general and with respect to sport competition in particular (Strahler *et al.*, 2010). The physiological response to stress or arousal is conceptualized as an individual's psychological and physiological autonomic system activation, varying on a continuum from deep sleep to extreme excitement (Gould and Krane, 1992). Whereas heart rate responds rapidly and non-specifically to perceived threats, most neuroendocrine effectors respond to specific stimuli, often with longer time courses. Neuroendocrine stress markers include catecholamines, such as adrenaline, noradrenaline and dopamine, as markers of the sympathetic adrenal medullary system (SAM), and cortisol as the primary marker of the hypothalamic–pituitary–adrenocortical axis (HPA axis). While it is clear that the HPA axis and the SAM work in coordination to generate the physiologic changes associated with the stress response, the exact nature of the coordination (e.g. additive or interactive; opposing or complementary) is a subject of debate.

Henry (1992) speculates that SAM activity increases in response to challenges that are perceived as manageable or controllable, whereas an HPA axis response is more likely during emotionally stressful or uncontrollable situations. The permissive, stimulatory, suppressive and preparative effects of HPA axis hormones released in response to stress are believed to ensure the maintenance of homeostasis through activation and coordination of various psychological and physiological processes, such as memory, immune functioning, cardiovascular activation, substrate metabolism, behavioural response to threatening circumstances and emotional processing (Sapolsky *et al.*, 2000; Erickson *et al.*, 2003).

For Gaab *et al.* (2005), the HPA axis is stimulated in anticipation of, or in response to a wide range of psychological stressors. The perception of threat would be the principal stimulus to induce HPA axis responses, while being strongly influenced by the perception of controllability. This is especially relevant in situations inducing ego-involvement, novelty and unpredictability, leading to negative affective states (Buchanan *et al.*, 1999). Besides the adaptive short- and medium-term consequences of acute stress-induced HPA axis responses, chronic dysregulation and/or excessive secretion of its hormones corticotrophin-releasing hormone (CRH), adrenocorticotrophin hormone (ACTH), and cortisol have been shown to exert detrimental effects on both somatic and mental well-being (Gaab *et al.*, 2005).

Studies investigating the neuroendocrine response to competition have mainly focused on the activity of the HPA axis. From an endocrinological point of view, the response to competitive situations is elicited even before the competitive activity starts. The organismic control of resources, including hormonal responses, in order to adjust to changing anticipated demands, has strongly been emphasized within the framework of the allostasis (Schulkin *et al.*, 1994). The existence of an anticipatory cortisol response prior to stressful events of a physical nature has long been recognized (Mason *et al.*, 1973). More recently, it has been reported that this anticipatory response to competition includes elevations of cortisol (Passelergue and Lac, 1999; Filaire *et al.*, 2001a) and of testosterone (Suay *et al.*, 1999). It has been suggested that this elevation of testosterone has a preparatory purpose, which is specific to competitive settings (Booth *et al.*, 1989). However, it has been pointed out that this anticipatory rise, while present in the aggregate, is not highly reliable across subjects. In several studies heightened testosterone before competitive situations has not been found (Passelergue and Lac, 1999; Filaire *et al.*, 2001b). A lower cortisol responsiveness following psychosocial stress has also been reported in trained compared to untrained men (Rimmele *et al.*, 2007, see Chapter 8), whereby the higher levels of self-efficacy and exercise-induced modulation in stress-responsiveness of the hormonal and autonomic system explain the reduced stress reactivity of trained men.

It has been stated that every anxiety-arousing situation is characterized by being perceived as a threat, by being only partially controlled, and by uncertainty about the outcome and/or its consequences (Sapolsky, 1994). Sport competition meets these three characteristics, including both physiological and psychosocial stressors. Hence, it can be considered as an anxiety-arousing situation. The different expectations and mood states prior to the contest could also play an important role in the hormonal anticipatory response. Some studies have shown that testosterone is positively associated with positive mood (vigour) assessed before competitive encounters (Salvador *et al.*, 2001), although another study failed to find a significant association with anxiety (Filaire *et al.*, 2001b).

In a general manner, there is a relationship between somatic and cognitive anxiety and cortisol (McKay *et al.*, 1997; Filaire *et al.*, 2001a), or by the direction of anxiety components and cortisol (Eubank *et al.*, 1997). Conversely, others studies found no relationship between anxiety intensity and cortisol concentrations before competition (Sight *et al.*, 1999; Thatcher *et al.*, 2004). Positive affective states seem to lower cortisol secretion (Frankenhaeuser, 1978). Mild increases in cortisol prepare individuals for action and lower cortisol concentrations may indicate more resilience to stressful situations (Stansbury and Gunnar, 1994; Kivlighan *et al.*, 2005). Increase in this hormone appears to be important in preparing for mental and physical demands, and may affect performance (Salvador *et al.*, 2003). However, extreme elevations in cortisol lead to poor performance because they interfere with some cognitive processes (Erickson *et al.*, 2003).

Competition has also been understood as a stressful situation in the animal and sport literature, where both the competition and its outcome are considered very significant stressors. For example, Eberhart *et al.* (1980) reported in several studies in non-human primates that a male's cortisol level changes when his status changes, rising when he achieves and falling when he is dominated. In humans, some researchers have analysed sport competitions, considering them socially acceptable situations where individuals compete in such a way that the encounters affect their sport status. However, the results are in debate. A number of studies have tried to confirm the differences in testosterone and cortisol response in humans, the differences depending on the outcome (victory or defeat), as found in other species. In this context, complex psychological processes related to emotional and/or cognitive interpretation of the situation have been claimed to be more important for hormonal responses than the outcome itself.

Recently, Salvador (2005) suggested integration of competition within a more general stress framework, considering that previous results on this topic can be better explained as a part of the coping response to competition. From this perspective, if the individual appraises the situation as important, controllable and depending on his or her effort, that is, if the person interprets the competitive situation as a challenge, an active coping response pattern is more likely to develop. This pattern would be characterized by increases in testosterone and sympathetic nervous system (SNS) activation, accompanied by positive mood changes, all of which would increase the probability of victory, although obviously it is not guaranteed. On the other hand, if the individual assesses the situation as threatening or uncontrollable, he or she will probably present a passive coping response pattern characterized by insufficient testosterone and SNS activation and increases in cortisol, accompanied by negative affect changes. This appraisal and the associated responses will increase the probability of defeat. In addition, the outcome finally obtained will be able to affect mood and satisfaction.

Obviously, the appraisal in a specific situation is the result of the interaction between many dimensions and variables, some probably not at conscious levels that have been mentioned throughout this review and others (Salvador and Costa, 2009). Moreover, the probability of success or lack of it associated with the response pattern will depend on the specific demands and processes involved in the specific competition in question. Finally, the emotions associated with the outcome obtained would depend on aspects such as the importance of the competition, motivation to win, status, etc. Thus, androgenic response has been associated with the involvement of the subject in the situation, with testosterone showing positive correlations with a motivation to win (Suay *et al.*, 1999), and internal attribution (Serrano *et al.*, 2000) but negative correlations with external attribution of the outcome (Gonzalez-Bono *et al.*, 1999). On the other hand, cortisol has been related to the state anxiety experienced during the contest (Serrano *et al.*, 2000).

Although the immediate cortisol response to competition is well established, longitudinal responses to competitive stress have hardly found any attention (Strahler *et al.*, 2010). Nevertheless, increases in cortisol across several competitions have been noted, which authors interpreted as a lack of habituation of the HPA axis activation to competitions (Rohleder *et al.*, 2007).

Recently, it has been suggested that the analysis of the cortisol awakening response (CAR) could be a potentially more interesting parameter than cortisol to explore longitudinal neuroendocrine reactions to competition stress. Numerous studies have suggested that the CAR serves as a marker of general HPA axis activity (see Clow *et al.*, 2004 for a review). On a physiological level, the CAR reflects the psychological anticipation of the demands of the respective day, higher anticipated demands leading to a higher CAR (Fries *et al.*, 2009). CAR can be assessed by taking saliva samples four to five times (usually every 15 minutes) during the first hour after awakening. Common parameters of the CAR used are not only the increase itself but also the released amount of cortisol, which can be calculated from the area under curve of the measurement time course. The CAR has been proven to be a distinct intra-individual reaction with a relative stability over time (Wüst *et al.*, 2000). Altered CAR has been noted to be linked to occupational stress (Federenko *et al.*, 2004) and mental health (Fries *et al.*, 2005). In contrast to daytime cortisol assessment, the CAR is not affected by physical stress, thereby constituting a valuable measure for the study of the longitudinal cortisol response to real-life stress events (Strahler *et al.*, 2010).

While there is evidence to suggest that this marker may represent a relatively stable, individual difference variable, there is also evidence to suggest that this cortisol response can be affected by gender. In fact, numerous studies have found greater CARs in women than in men (Clow *et al.*, 2004). Sex differences in CAR were also found during (higher stress) workdays, with females demonstrating greater CARs than men (Kunz-Ebrecht *et al.*, 2004; Filaire *et al.*, 2009).

Data in the literature also suggest a possible age-related shift in gender differences. At younger ages, numerous studies have suggested that males demonstrate greater levels of cortisol in response to stressors than do females. However, the vast majority of these studies have been performed using laboratory stressors. Moreover, it seems that the nature of the gender difference is complex, and in sport, for example, the level of competitive experience, the specific phase of the competitive event and the social affiliation with team-mates also affect these gender differences (Kivlighan *et al.*, 2005).

The physiological response to psychological stressors consists also of an activation of the sympathetic nervous system (SNS), a parasympathetic withdrawal. Direct measurements of adrenaline and noradrenaline in saliva do not seem to reflect sympathoadrenal medulla (SAM) activity (Schwab *et al.*, 1992). Salivary alpha-amylase (sAA) concentrations have been suggested as an indirect marker for SAM activity under a variety of stressful conditions (Bosch *et al.*, 2003; Nater *et al.*, 2005; Kivlighan and Granger, 2006). However, this marker is in debate. In fact, in early studies sAA activity emerged as a measure of parasympathetic activity, whereby sAA levels were found to increase during relaxation (Morse *et al.*, 1983). The mid-1990s, however, saw the first studies showing that sAA activity is increased during stress and correlates with noradrenaline release during exercise.

Alpha-amylase is produced by the serous acinar cells of the parotid and submandibular glands. It is one of the principal salivary proteins appearing as a number of isoenzymes. Amylase accounts for 10–20% of the total salivary gland-produced protein content and is mostly synthesized by the parotid gland (see Chapter 6). Kivlighan and Granger (2006) reported that sAA changes in response to, but not in anticipation of competition. It is important to note that stress-related changes in AA and cortisol concentrations do not appear to correlate (Nater *et al.*, 2006). Other stress studies report that changes in sAA activity do not, or only modestly, correlate with changes in other SNS markers, such as cardiac pre-ejection period, skin conductance and plasma noradrenaline. Even within the salivary glands, the SNS does not act in a concerted fashion: the secreto-motor sympathetic nerve fibres responsible for the glandular secretion of sAA are activated independently of the vasoconstriction in glandular tissue (Proctor and Carpenter, 2007).

Recently, Bosch *et al.* (2011) have discussed a number of common misconceptions and methodological issues that surround the use of sAA as a marker of SNS activity and conclude that at present there is insufficient support for the use and interpretation of sAA activity as a valid and reliable measure of SNS activity.

For monitoring the activity of the SNS salivary chromogranin A (CgA) has also been demonstrated to be a valid quantitative index (Nakane *et al.*, 1998). CgA is a soluble protein that is stored and co-released by exocytosis with catecholamines from the adrenal medulla and sympathetic nerve endings. Dimsdale *et al.* (1992) reported that the plasma CgA level correlates with the noradrenaline release rate. This result indicates that the plasma CgA level may be an index of the activity of the sympathetic/adrenomedullary system. Salivary CgA was shown to be produced by the human submandibular gland and secreted into saliva (Saruta *et al.*, 2005), and is considered to be a sensitive and reliable index for evaluating psychological stress. Yanaihura *et al.* (1998) found that salivary CgA is a sensitive marker of the initial psychological phase of the stress response and some papers reported a rapid and sensitive elevation of salivary CgA in response to such psychosomatic stressors as public speaking and driving a car (Nakane *et al.*, 1998; Nakane *et al.*, 2002). Therefore, these salivary biomarkers may be useful indicators for assessing mental stress. However, to our knowledge there are no studies of precompetitive anxiety in relation to this biomarker.

Conclusion and future indications

Anxiety is widely regarded as a complex psychological phenomenon, and is probably one of the most difficult emotions to define and diagnose. In sport psychology, the theoretical relationship between competitive anxiety and sports performance has been one of the most debated and investigated domains (Woodman and Hardy, 2001). From an endocrinological point of view, the response to competitive situations is elicited even before the competitive activity starts, and stimulates the activity of the HPA axis and SAM. These neuroendocrine responses can be evaluated through non-invasive biomarkers. The association between anticipatory hormonal responses and psychological dimensions is not clear, but instead shows results suggesting a fairly complex description of relationships. Novel directions of future research need address the question concerning whether the reduced basal HPA axis activity in trained men, as found by Rimmele *et al.* (2007) and Strahler *et al.* (2010), is due to competitions or extensive physical exercise or to both.

A second direction should follow the consideration that the HPA axis response to competition could be moderated by competitive trait anxiety. Similarly, in addition to assessing the intensity of anxiety symptoms, the frequency of occurrence of these symptoms and the direction of their interpretation should be considered. In general, further studies using non-invasive markers and in particular the cortisol awakening response and salivary CgA and sAA evolution in sport competitions are needed to better understand the relationship between emotion, behaviour, hormones and performance.

Moreover, the salivary dehydroepiandrosterone (DHEA) response to situations causing social anxiety, as is the case in competition, seems to be of some interest. In fact, DHEA, in addition to cortisol, is a major steroid produced by the zona reticularis of the adrenal cortex, and recent findings have implicated it in the regulation of mental states. However, the mechanism of stress-induced DHEA secretion and DHEA reactivity to psychosocial stimuli has not been sufficiently understood, especially in sport.

References

Apter, M. (1982). *The Experience of Motivation: The Theory of Psychological Reversals*. New York: Academic Press.

Booth, A., Shelley, G., Mazur, A., Tharp, G. and Kittok, R. (1989). Testosterone and winning and losing in human competition. *Hormones and Behavior*, 23, 556–571.

Bosch, J. A., de Geus, E. J., Veerman, E. C., Hoogstaten, J. and Nieuw Amerongen, A. V.

(2003). Innate secretory immunity in response to laboratory stressors that evoke distinct patterns of cardiac autonomic activity. *Psychosomatic Medicine*, 65, 245–258.

Bosch, J. A., Veerman, E. C. I., de Geus J. and Proctor, G. B. (2011). Alpha-amylase as a reliable and convenient measure of sympathetic activity: don't start salivating just yet. *Psychoneuroendocrinology*, 36, 449–453.

Buchanan, T. W., al'Absi, M. and Lovallo, W. R. (1999). Cortisol fluctuates with increases and decreases in negative affect. *Psychoneuroendocrinology*, 24, 227–241.

Cheng, W. N. K, Hardy, L. and Markland, D. (2009). Toward a three-dimensional conceptualization of performance anxiety: Rationale and initial measurement development. *Psychology of Sport and Exercise*, 10, 271–278.

Cheng, W. N. K., Hardy, L. and Woodman, T. (2011). Predictive validity of a three-dimensional model of performance anxiety in the context of tae-kwon-do. *Journal of Sport and Exercise Psychology*, 33, 40–53.

Clow, A., Evans, T. and Hucklebridge, F. (2004). The awakening cortisol response: methodological issues and significance. *Stress*, 7, 29–37.

Dimsdale, J. E., O'Connor, D. T., Ziegler, M. and Mills, P. (1992). Chromogranin A correlates with norepinephrine release rate. *Life Sciences*, 51, 519–525.

Eberhart, J. A., Keverne, E. B. and Meller, R. E. (1980). Social influences on plasma testosterone levels in male talapoin monkeys. *Hormones and Behavior*, 14, 247–266.

Edward, T. and Hardy, L. (1996). The interactive effects of intensity and direction of cognitive and somatic anxiety and self-confidence upon performance. *Journal of Sport and Exercise Psychology*, 18, 296–312.

Erickson, K., Drevets, W. and Schulkin, J. (2003). Glucocorticoid regulation of diverse cognitive functions in normal and pathological emotional states. *Neurosciences and Biobehavioral Review*, 27, 233–246.

Eubank, M., Collins, D., Lovell, G., Dorling, D. and Talbot, S. (1997). Individual temporal differences in pre-competition anxiety and hormonal concentration. *Personality and Individual Differences*, 23, 1031–1039.

Federenko, I., Wüst, S., Hellhammer, D. H., Dechoux, R., Kumsta, R. and Kirschbaum, C. (2004). Free cortisol awakening responses are influenced by awakening time. *Psychoneuroendocrinology*, 29, 174–184.

Filaire, E., Sagnol, M., Ferrand, C. and Lac, G. (2001a). Psychophysiological stress in judo athletes during competitions. *Journal of Sports Medicine and Physical Fitness*, 41, 263–268.

Filaire, E., Maso, F., Sagnol, M., Le Scanff, C. and Lac, G. (2001b). Anxiety, hormonal responses, and coping during a judo competition. *Aggressive Behavior*, 27, 55–63.

Filaire, E., Alix, D., Ferrand, C. and Verger, M. (2009). Psychophysiological stress in tennis players during the first single match of a tournament. *Psychoneuroendocrinology*, 34, 150–157.

Fletcher, D. and Fletcher, J. (2005). A meta-model of stress, emotions and performance: conceptual foundations, theoretical framework, and research directions. *Journal of Sports Sciences*, 2, 157–158.

Frankenhaeuser, M. (1978). Psychoneuroendocrine approaches to the study of emotion as related to stress and coping. *Nebraska Symposium of Motivation*, 26, 123–161.

Fries, E., Hesse, J., Hellhammer, J. and Hellhammer, D. H. (2005). A new view on hypocortisolism. *Psychoneuroendocrinology*, 30, 1010–1016.

Fries, E., Dettenborn, L. and Kirschbaum, C. (2009). The cortisol awakening response (CAR): facts and future direction. *International Journal of Psychophysiology*, 72, 67–73.

Gaab, J., Rohlede, N., Nater, U. M. and Ehlert, U. (2005). Psychological determinants of the cortisol stress response: the role of anticipatory cognitive appraisal. *Psychoneuroendocrinology*, 30, 599–610.

Gonzalez-Bono, E., Salvador, A., Serrano, M. A. and Ricarte, J. (1999). Testosterone, cortisol, and mood in a sports team competition. *Hormones and Behavior*, 35, 55–62.

Gould, D. and Krane, V. (1992). The arousal-athletic performance relationship: current status and future directions. In T. S. Horn (ed.), *Advances in Sport Psychology* (pp. 142–149). Champaign, IL: Human Kinetics.

Gould, D., Greenleaf, C. and Krane, V. (2002). Arousal-anxiety and sport behavior. In T. S. Horn (ed.), *Advances in Sport Psychology* (pp. 207–241). Champaign, IL: Human Kinetics.

Hanin, Y. L. (1995). Individual zones of optimal functioning (IZOF) model: an idiographic approach to performance anxiety. In K. Henschen and W. Straub (eds), *Sport Psychology: An Analysis of Athlete Behavior* (pp. 103–199). Longmeadow, NY: Mouvement.

Hanin, Y. L. (2007). Emotions in sport: current issues and perspectives. In G. Tenenbaum and R. C. Eklund (eds), *Handbook of Sport Psychology*, 3rd edn. pp. 31–58). Hoboken, NJ: Wiley.

Hardy, L. (1996). A test of catastrophe models of anxiety and sports performance against multidimensional anxiety theory models using the method of dynamic differences. *Anxiety, Stress, and Coping*, 9, 69–86.

Hardy, L., Jones, G. and Gould, D. (1996). *Understanding Psychological Preparation for Sport: Theory and Practice of Elite Performers*. Chichester: Wiley.

Hatfield, B. D. and Landers, D. M. (1983). Psychophysiology: a new direction for sport psychology. *Journal of Sport Psychology*, 5, 243–259.

Henry, J. P. (1992). Biological basis of the stress response. *Integrative Physiological and Behavioral Science*, 27, 66–83.

Jones, G. (1995). More than just a game: research developments and issues in competitive anxiety in sport. *British Journal of Psychology*, 86, 449–478.

Jones, G. (1991). Recent issues in competitive state anxiety research. *The Psychologist*, 4, 152–155.

Jones, G. and Hanton, S. (2001). Pre-competitive feeling states and directional anxiety interpretations. *Journal of Sports Sciences*, 19, 385–395.

Jones, G. and Swain, A. B. (1992). Intensity and direction dimensions of competitive state anxiety and relationships with competitiveness. *Perceptual and Motor Skills*, 74, 467–472.

Jones, G., Swain, A. and Hardy, L. (1993). Intensity and direction dimensions of competitive state anxiety and relationships with performance. *Journal of Sport Sciences*, 11, 525–532.

Jones, M., Meijn, C., McCarthy, P. J. and Sheffield, D. (2009). A theory of challenge and threat states in athletes. *International Review of Sport and Exercise Psychology*, 2, 161–180.

Kerr, J. H. (1997). *Motivation and Emotion in Sport: Reversal Theory*. Methuen: Psychology Press.

Kivilighan, K. T. and Granger, D. (2006). Salivary alpha-amylase response to competition: relation to gender, previous experience, and attitudes. *Psychoneuroendocrinology*, 31, 703–714.

Kivlighan, K. T, Granger, D. A. and Booth, A. (2005). Gender differences in testosterone and cortisol response to competition. *Psychoneuroendocrinology*, 30, 58–71.

Kunz-Ebrecht, S. R., Kirschbaum, C., Marmot, M. and Steptoe, A. (2004). Differences in cortisol awakening responses on work days and weekends in women and men from the Whitehall II cohort. *Psychoneuroendocrinology*, 29, 516–528.

Landers, D. M. (1980). The arousal-performance relationship revisited. *Research Quarterly for Exercise and Sport*, 51, 77–90.

Lazarus, R. S. (1981). The stress and coping paradigm. In C. Eisdorfer, D. Cohen, A. Kleinman and P. Maxim (eds), *Models for Clinical Psychopathology* (pp. 177–224). New York: Spectrum.

Lazarus, R. S. and Folkman, S. (1986). Cognitive theories of stress and the issue of circularity. In M. H. Appley and R. Trumbull (eds), *Dynamics of Stress. Physiological, Psychological, and Social Perspectives* (pp. 63–80). New York: Plenum Press.

Martens, R., Vealey, R. S. and Burton, D. (1990). *Competitive Anxiety in Sport*. Champaign, IL: Human Kinetics.

Mason, J. W., Hartley, L. H., Kotchen, T. A., Mougey, E. H., Ricketts, P. T. and Jones, L. G. (1973). Plasma cortisol and norepinephrine responses in anticipation of muscular exercise. *Psychosomatic Medicine*, 35, 406–414.

McEwen, B. S. (1998). Protective and damaging effects of stress. *New England Journal of Medicine*, 338, 171–179.

McEwen, B. S., Sakai, R. R. and Spencer, R. L. (1993). Adrenal steroid effects on the brain: versatile hormones with good and bad effects. In J. Schulkin (ed.), *Hormonally Induced Changes in Mind and Brain* (pp. 157–189). San Diego, CA: Academic Press.

McKay, J. M., Selig, S. E., Carlson, J. S. and Morris, T. (1997). Psychophysiological stress in elite golfers during practice and competition. *Australian Journal of Science and Medicine in Sport*, 29, 55–61.

Melallieu, S., Hanton, S. and Fletcher, D. (2009). *A Competitive Anxiety Review: Directions in Sport Psychology Research*. New York: Nova Science Publishers.

Morris, L. W. and Liebert, R. M. (1973). Effects of negative feedback, threat of shock, and trait anxiety on the arousal of two components of anxiety. *Journal of Educational Psychology*, 20, 321–326.

Morse, D. R., Schacterle, G. R., Furst, M. L., Esposito, J. V. and Zaydenburg, M. (1983). Stress, relaxation and saliva: relationship to dental caries and its prevention, with a literature review. *Annals of Dentistry*, 42, 47–54.

Nakane, H., Asami, O., Yamada, Y., Harada, T., Matsui, N. and Kanno, T. (1998). Salivary chromogranin A as an index of psychosomatic stress response. *Biomedical Research*, 18, 401–406.

Nakane, H., Asami, O., Yamada, Y. and Ohira, H. (2002). Effect of negative air ions on computer operation, anxiety and salivary chromogranin A-like immunoreactivity. *International Journal of Psychophysiology*, 46, 85–89.

Nater, U. M., Rohleder, N., Gaab, J., *et al.* (2005). Human salivary alpha-amylase reactivity in a psychosocial stress paradigm. *International Journal of Psychophysiology*, 55, 333–342.

Nater, U. M., La Marca, R., Florin, L., *et al.* (2006). Stress-induced changes in human salivary alpha-amylase activity-associations with adrenergic activity. *Psychoneuroendocrinology*, 31, 49–58.

Passelergue, P. and Lac, G. (1999). Saliva cortisol, testosterone and T/C ratio variations during a wrestling competition and during the post-competitive recovery period. *International Journal of Sports Medicine*, 20, 109–113.

Proctor, G. B. and Carpenter, G. H. (2007). Regulation of salivary gland function by autonomic nerves. *Autonomic Neuroscience*, 133, 3–18.

Rimmele, U., Zellweger, B. C., Marti, B., *et al.* (2007). Trained men show lower cortisol, heart rate and psychological responses to psychosocial stress compared with untrained men. *Psychoneuroendocrinology*, 32, 627–635.

Rohleder, N., Beulen, S. E., Chen, E., Wolf, J. M. and Kirschbaum, C. (2007). Stress on the dance floor: the cortisol response to social-evaluative threat in competitive ballroom dancers. *Personality and Social Psychology Bulletin*, 33, 69–84.

Salvador, A. (2005). Coping with competitive situations in humans. *Neurosciences and Biobehavioral Reviews*, 29, 195–205.

Salvador, A. and Costa, R. (2009). Coping with competition: neuroendocrine responses and cognitive variables. *Neurosciences and Biobehavioral Reviews*, 33, 160–170.

Salvador, A., Ricarte, J., González-Bono, E. and Moya-Albiol, L. (2001). Effects of physical training on endocrine and autonomic responsiveness to acute stress. *Journal of Psychophysiology*, 15, 114–121.

Salvador, A., Suay, F., Gonzalez-Bono, E. and Serrano, M. A. (2003). Anticipatory cortisol, testosterone and psychological responses to judo competition in young men. *Psychoneuroendocrinology*, 28, 364–375.

Sapolsky, R. M. (1994) *Why Zebras Don't Get Ulcers: An Updated Guide to Stress, Stress-related Diseases, and Coping.* New York: WH Freeman

Sapolsky, R. M., Romero, L. M. and Munck, A. U. (2000). How do glucocorticoids influence stress responses? Integrating permissive, suppressive, stimulatory, and preparative actions. *Endocrinology Review*, 21, 55–89.

Saruta, J., Tsukinoki, K., Sasaguri, K., *et al.* (2005). Expression and localization of chromogranin A, purification and characterization from catecholamine storage vesicles of human pheochromocytoma. *Hypertension*, 6, 2–12.

Schulkin, J., McEwen, B. S. and Gold, P. W. (1994). Allostasis, amygdala and anticipatory angst. *Neuroscience and Biobehavioral Reviews*, 18, 385–396.

Schwab, K. O., Heubel, G. and Bartels, H. (1992). Free epinephrine, norepinephrine and dopamine in saliva and plasma of healthy adults. *European Journal of Clinical Chemistry and Clinical Biochemistry*, 30, 541–544.

Serrano, M. A., Salvador, A., Gonzalez-Bono, E., Sanchis, C. and Suay, F. (2000). Hormonal responses to competition: do outcome, effort, mood or attribution matter? *Psicothema*, 12, 440–444.

Sight, A., Petrides, J. S., Gold, P., Chrousos, G. and Deuster, P. (1999). Differential hypothalamic-pituitary-adrenal axis reactivity to psychological and physical stress. *Journal of Endocrinology and Metabolism*, 84, 1944–1948.

Smith, R. E., Smoll, F. L., Cumming, S. P. and Grossbard, J. R. (2006). Measurement of multidimensional sport performance anxiety in children and adults: the sport anxiety scale-2. *Journal of Sport and Exercise Psychology*, 28, 479–501.

Stansbury, K. and Gunnar, M. (1994). Adrenocortical activity and emotion regulation. *Monographs of the Society for Research in Child Development*, 59, 108–134.

Sterling, P. and Eyer, E. (1988). Allostasis: a new paradigm to explain arousal pathology. In S. Fisher and J. Reason (eds), *Handbook of Life Stress, Cognition and Health* (pp. 629–649). New York: Wiley.

Strahler, K., Ehrlenspiel, F., Heene, M. and Brand, R. (2010). Competitive anxiety and cortisol awakening response in the week leading up to a competition. *Psychology of Sport and Exercise*, 11, 148–154.

Suay, F., Salvador, A., Gonzalez-Bono, E., Sanchis, C., Martinez, M., Martinez-Sanchis, S., *et al.* (1999). Effects on competition and its outcome on serum testosterone, cortisol and prolactin. *Psychoneuroendocrinology*, 24, 551–566.

Swain, A. B. J. and Jones, G. (1993). Intensity and frequency dimensions of competitive state anxiety. *Journal of Sports Sciences*, 11, 533–542.

Thatcher, J., Thatcher, R. and Dorling, D. (2004). Gender differences in the pre-competition temporal patterning of anxiety and hormonal responses. *Journal of Sport Medicine and Physical Fitness*, 44, 300–308.

Woodman, T. and Hardy, L. (2001). Stress and anxiety. In R. Singer, H. A. Hausenblas and C. M. Janelle (eds), *Handbook of Research on Sport Psychology* (pp. 290–318). New York: Wiley.

Wüst, S., Wolf, J., Hellhammer, D. H., Federenko, I., Schommer, N. and Kirschbaum, C. (2000). The cortisol awakening response-normal values and confounds. *Noise and Health*, 7, 77–85.

Yanaihura, N., Nishikawa, Y. and Hoshino, M. (1998). Evaluation of region-specific radioimmunoassays for rat and human chromogranin A: measurement of immunoreactivity in plasma, urine and saliva. In T. Kanno, Y. Nakazato and K. Kumakura (eds), *The Adrenal Chromaffin Cell* (pp. 305–313). Sapporo: Hokkaido University Press.

8 Physical activity and psychophysiological stress reactivity

Ulrike Rimmele

Physical activity has proven benefits for physical and psychological well-being and is associated with reduced responsiveness to physical stress. However, it is not clear to what extent physical activity also modulates responsiveness to psychosocial stress. Here a research programme is presented that tests whether and how physical activity modulates hormonal, cardiovascular and subjective psychological responses to a psychosocial stressor. The presented research allows a better understanding of the preventive role of physical activity in stress responsiveness and can be taken as a foundation for intervention studies in healthy and clinical populations.

Physical activity, stress and stress-related disorders

Physical activity is commonly regarded as beneficial to both physical and psychological health, and is seen as an effective preventive measure and treatment for the detrimental consequences of chronic stress and stress-related diseases, such as cardiovascular disorders or depression (Steptoe *et al.*, 1993; Babyak *et al.*, 2000; Talbot *et al.*, 2002; Ketelhut *et al.*, 2004; Motl *et al.*, 2004). Physically active people show reduced reactivity to physical stressors as well as reduced susceptibility to the adverse influences of life stress (Deuster *et al.*, 1989; Dishman, 1997; Throne *et al.*, 2000; Dishman *et al.*, 2006; Rimmele *et al.*, 2007). Moreover, it has been proposed that physical activity influences stress reactivity more generally, with protective effects also when confronted with non-physical stressors (e.g. mental stress) (Claytor, 1991; Cox, 1991; Sothmann *et al.*, 1991, 1996).

Since non-physical stressors, such as psychosocial stressors, increase the risk of developing cardiovascular and mental diseases, such as hypertension or depression (Gold *et al.*, 1988; McEwen, 2002; Vanitallie, 2002), it is important to assess whether physical activity may reduce the responsiveness to psychosocial stressors, thereby contributing to the prevention of stress-related disorders with major public health significance (McEwen, 1998).

Employing a cross-stressor adaptation hypothesis (Selye, 1950), several researchers have argued that the adaptation of the stress systems as a result of physical activity may not only influence physiological stress reactivity to physical stress, but also to non-exercise stress, such as psychological stress (de Geus *et al.*, 1990; Sothmann *et al.*, 1996). The cross-stressor adaptation hypothesis is grounded in the fact that the physiological reactivity to both physical and psychological stressors leads to an activation of the sympathetic nervous system (SNS) and hypothalamic–pituitary–adrenal (HPA) axis (Luger *et al.*, 1987; Deuster *et al.*, 1989; Kirschbaum *et al.*, 1993; Dickerson and Kemeny, 2004). Activation of the SNS changes the activation status of the cardiovascular, respiratory, gastrointestinal, renal and other systems (Cacioppo *et al.*, 1998; McEwen, 2000; Tsigos and Chrousos, 2002). For example, blood pressure and heart rate rise, and the lungs expand. Also due to activation of the SNS, blood transport to the muscles is promoted and eye and hair follicle muscles are activated. This explains why stressed individuals display eyes wide open and hair standing on end. These physiological reactions are mediated in two ways: (1) by direct activation of sympathetic nerves affecting adrenergic receptors on their target organs via nerve fibres secreting noradrenaline, and (2) by indirect activation involving the sympathetic adrenal medullary (SAM) system (Tsigos and Chrousos, 2002).

In addition, stressors affect HPA axis activity (Tsigos and Chrousos, 2002). As a result, three key hormones are released, one on each level of the HPA axis (Tsigos and Chrousos, 2002): (1) corticotrophin-releasing hormone (CRH), (2) adrenocorticotrophin hormone (ACTH), and (3) a species-specific glucocorticoid (cortisol in humans) (Tsigos and Chrousos, 2002). Following chronic stress, alterations in these systems have been linked to the development of stress-related disorders (McEwen, 1998; Steptoe, 1991). Since stress-related diseases cost a considerable amount to economies and healthcare systems (Kalia, 2002), potential protective factors against the development of stress-related disorders are sought. Physical activity, with its beneficial effects on physiological stress systems, has long been proposed as such a protective factor against stress and stress-related disorders.

Chronic exercise is associated with numerous biological adaptations that result in efficient physiological functioning. These adaptations include changes in maximum oxygen uptake, heart rate, heart size, onset of lactate production and hormonal regulation. These physiological adaptations moderate the physiological response to physical stressors and permit trained subjects to cope more efficiently with physical stressors (Petruzzello *et al.*, 1997). For example, physically active individuals have been found to exhibit an attenuated HPA and sympathetic reactivity, including lower heart rate reactivity and greater heart rate recovery to physical stressors compared with untrained individuals (Luger *et al.*, 1987; Deuster *et al.*, 1989; Moya-Albiol *et al.*, 2001). This adaptation of stress-responsive systems due to exercise may influence stress responses not only to physical stressors but also to psychological stressors, such as mental stressors (Claytor, 1991; Cox, 1991; Sothmann *et al.*, 1996; Sothmann *et al.*, 1991), and crucially such as psychosocial stressors. Based on this background, physical activity may be a general protective factor against different kinds of stressors.

Considering that psychosocial stressors are more relevant in today's societies than physical stressors, but the physiological stress regulation systems have mainly evolved to deal with acute physical stressors, it is especially relevant to understand how the physiological responses to psychosocial stress, which may often be inadequate, can be influenced. However, both cross-sectional and longitudinal studies, which have sought to determine the influence of physical activity on reactivity to psychological stressors have reported inconsistent findings (de Geus and van Doornen, 1993).

A comprehensive meta-analytic review of 34 studies by Crews and Landers (1987) on the relationship between aerobic fitness and reactivity to psychosocial stressors found an average effect size estimate of 0.48 ($P < 0.01$), suggesting that aerobically fit subjects have lower stress reactivity compared to baseline values or control group values (Crews and Landers, 1987). Later studies confirmed such lower psychophysiological responses to psychological stressors in groups of men with different degrees of physical activity using several psychophysiological measures (Boutcher and Landers, 1988; Steptoe *et al.*, 1990; Moya-Albiol *et al.*, 2001; Spalding *et al.*, 2004). However, some studies included in the meta-analysis by Crews and Landers, as well as reviews of longitudinal studies (de Geus and van Doornen, 1993), reported non-significant findings between exercise/fitness and stress reactivity or higher stress reactivity in aerobically fit subjects (Crews and Landers, 1987; de Geus *et al.*, 1993). Furthermore, evidence from 73 studies in a meta-regression analysis that examined the influence of fitness on cardiovascular responses during and after acute laboratory stress in humans indicates that fitness is associated with slightly greater stress reactivity, but better recovery (Jackson and Dishman, 2006).

Most studies that have investigated the relationship between fitness and psychosocial stress response compared trained and untrained subjects, using inactive men as a control group (Sinyor *et al.*, 1983; Crews and Landers, 1987; Claytor *et al.*, 1988; Steptoe *et al.*, 1993), whereas a few employed a longitudinal experimental design (Claytor, 1991; de Geus and van Doornen, 1993; Senkfor and Williams, 1995; Spalding *et al.*, 2004). Also, fitness was differently defined and measured in these studies. Some studies used ergonometry tests and assessed maximal oxygen uptake to determine fitness levels, while other studies relied on self-reported training levels. Aside from fitness levels, studies also differed in sample size and the sex of subjects. Furthermore, the studies used various kinds of stressors and thus there was a lack of standardization in this dimension (Claytor, 1991; Jackson and Dishman, 2006). Most studies employed mental stressors based on cognitive performance, while others used passive stressors such as viewing film clips (Hull *et al.*, 1984). Designs also varied in the parameters that were used to assess stress reactivity. Most studies focused on assessing physiological variables, above cardiovascular changes. Whereas some studies reported blunted cardiovascular responses or a more rapid recovery in trained men (Holmes and Roth, 1985; Sinyor *et al.*, 1983, 1986; Crews and Landers, 1987; Boutcher and Landers, 1988; Steptoe *et al.*, 1990; Moya-Albiol *et al.*, 2001; Spalding *et al.*, 2004), others were unable to confirm such effects, or even reported higher reactivity (de Geus and van Doornen, 1993; Jackson and Dishman, 2006). In comparison to cardiovascular indicators of stress reactivity, few studies investigated stress reactivity by assessment of changes in hormonal levels, such as catecholamine or cortisol levels in urine, blood or saliva (Claytor, 1991; Sothmann *et al.*, 1991; Moyna *et al.*, 1999; Moya-Albiol *et al.*, 2001).

With regard to hormonal responses to stress, some studies found no effect of fitness on noradrenaline and adrenaline levels in plasma or urine (Brooke and Long, 1987; Claytor *et al.*, 1988; de Geus *et al.*, 1993), while others reported higher noradrenaline levels in plasma in trained subjects early on in the stress period (Sinyor *et al.*, 1983). In contrast, some studies found lower levels of fitness to be associated with an augmented noradrenaline response (Sothmann *et al.*, 1991; Moyna *et al.*, 1999). Notably, studies on HPA axis reactivity to psychological stressors did not show significant effects of physical fitness on cortisol levels (Sinyor *et al.*, 1983; Moyna *et al.*, 1999). With regard to psychological responses to stress, only nine out of 34 studies assessed psychological responses in the meta-analysis by Crews and Landers (1987). For example, Sinyor *et al.* (1983) found aerobically fit subjects to exhibit lower state anxiety following a psychological stressor.

In sum, it appears that being physically active may differentially influence an individual's reactivity to psychosocial stress depending on the kind and intensity of physical activity, the level of physical fitness, the age and gender of the subjects, the method of measurement, the time of day of stress induction and the type of stressor. It might be the case that the previous studies (Sinyor *et al.*, 1983; Moyna *et al.*, 1999) used stressors with low social impact. Since social evaluation has been found to be a strong trigger for an increase in cortisol responses (Biondi and Picardi, 1999), using a stressor with low social impact might have prevented different HPA responses in physically trained versus untrained subjects. However a stressor that includes a social-evaluative situation inducing a strong cortisol response (Biondi and Picardi, 1999) has barely been used to investigate the stress response of trained men. Thus it is not clear to what extent physical activity also modulates responsiveness to psychosocial stress.

Empirical studies on physical activity and psychophysiological stress reactivity

In the research presented here, we used the standardized Trier Social Stress Test (TSST), which enables a naturalistic exposure to a socio-evaluative stressful situation. The TSST comprises a 5-minute public speaking task followed by a 5-minute mental arithmetic task in front of an unknown panel of one man and one woman. In addition a video camera records the performance on the stress test. During the 5-minute speaking task, participants are instructed to give a mock job interview. The mental arithmetic task consists of counting backwards aloud (e.g. backwards from 1024 in steps of 13). The TSST has been shown to lead to two- to threefold increases in HPA axis and cardiovascular responses, as well as changes in psychological states (e.g. changes in mood, calmness and anxiety) (Kirschbaum *et al.*, 1993, 1999; Heinrichs *et al.*, 2001; Dickerson and Kemeny, 2004). Notably, it has been found to be the socio-evaluative character of the TSST that is crucial for the robust stress response (Dickerson and Kemeny, 2004).

Since differences in stress reactivity should be most evident when contrasting results from extreme groups of physical activity levels, in the research programme presented here, we first compared the stress responses of elite athletes with that of untrained men to test whether and how physical activity may modulate hormonal, cardiovascular and subjective responses to a psychosocial stressor. In a second study we tested how different levels of physical activity may modulate stress reactivity to a psychosocial stressor and examined whether moderator variables such as competitiveness play a role herein.

Lower responsiveness to psychosocial stress in elite athletes

In a first study, we compared the physiological and psychological reactivity to a psychosocial stressor of 22 healthy male elite athletes to the stress reactivity of 22 untrained healthy young men.

Methods

Elite sportsmen were primarily recruited from endurance-trained sports and had a Swiss Olympic Card and/or were members of the Swiss national teams. Untrained men exercised for less than 2 hours per week. Elite athletes and untrained men did not significantly differ in terms of age (athletes: 21.5 ± 2.35 years, untrained men: 21.84 ± 2.24), and body mass index (athletes: 23.2 ± 1.9, untrained men: 23.3 ± 3.2). Participants were ineligible if they were using medication or reported any mental or medical illness. Psychological symptoms were assessed with the Symptom Checklist (SCL-90-R, Global Severity Index). Further exclusion criteria were smoking more than five cigarettes per day and increased levels of chronic stress assessed with the Perceived Stress Scale (Cohen *et al.*, 1983).

Psychosocial stress was induced by the TSST (Kirschbaum *et al.*, 1993). In order to ensure high ego-involvement, elite athletes and untrained men were confronted with subjectively important situations. Elite athletes were instructed to apply for a contract with a sponsor and untrained men were asked to convince the audience that they were the most suitable person for a job of their choice. Under both conditions, the panel of evaluators was presented as experts in evaluating non-verbal behaviour. In addition, the panel of evaluators was instructed not to provide any visual or verbal feedback with the exception that, whenever the participant made a mistake in the mental arithmetic task, he was instructed to start from the beginning.

After entering the TSST room, subjects remained in a standing position throughout the 10-minute stress protocol. Following completion of the stress session, all participants were instructed to rest quietly for 90 minutes until saliva sampling was completed. Adrenocortical and autonomic responses to psychosocial stress were assessed by repeated measures of salivary free cortisol levels and heart rate. Salivary free cortisol has been found to be highly correlated with the unbound cortisol concentration in plasma and is considered to be a reliable and valid indicator of the biologically active fraction of cortisol (Vining *et al.*, 1983; Kirschbaum and Hellhammer, 1989, 1994). Heart rate was monitored at 5-second intervals throughout the experiment using a wireless chest heart rate transmitter and a wrist monitor recorder (Polar S810i; Polar Electro, Finland). Psychological responses before and after stress exposure were repeatedly assessed with two questionnaires: the state scale of the State-Trait Anxiety Inventory (Spielberger *et al.*, 1970) measured state anxiety responses to the stressor and the Multidimensional Mood Questionnaire (Steyer *et al.*, 1997) assessed mood and calmness.

Results

The psychosocial stress protocol induced significant increases in salivary free cortisol levels (Figure 8.1) and heart rate (Figure 8.2) in both elite athletes and untrained men. Crucially, the elite athletes showed significantly lower cortisol and heart rate increases in response to the stressor compared with the group of untrained men, while cortisol levels and heart rate did not differ between both groups at baseline. The stressor also affected psychological parameters in both elite athletes and untrained men: state anxiety increased and mood worsened (Figure 8.3). Following the stress protocol untrained men had higher state anxiety and worse mood than elite athletes, even though these parameters had not been different at baseline between elite athletes and untrained men. Interestingly, elite athletes also demonstrated higher calmness levels compared to untrained men throughout the experimental session.

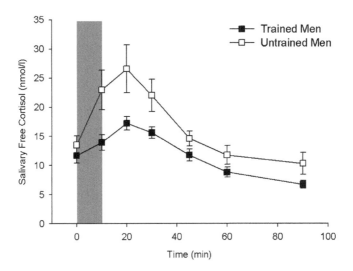

Figure 8.1 Mean salivary free cortisol levels before, during and after a standardized psychosocial stressor (Trier Social Stress Test) in trained and untrained men. The shaded area indicates the 10-minute period of stress exposure. Error bars are standard errors of the mean (SEM). Reprinted from Rimmele *et al.* (2007). Trained men showed lower cortisol, heart rate and psychological responses to psychosocial stress compared with untrained men. *Psychoneuroendocrinology*, 32, 627–635. Copyright (2007), with permission from Elsevier.

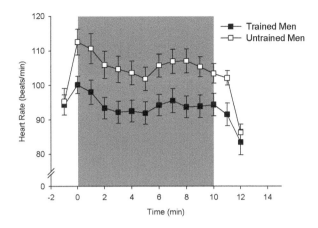

Figure 8.2 Mean heart rates before, during (shaded area) and after the Trier Social Stress
Test in trained and untrained men. Error bars are standard errors of the mean
(SEM). Reprinted from Rimmele *et al.* (2007). Trained men show lower cortisol, heart rate and psychological responses to psychosocial stress compared with
untrained men. *Psychoneuroendocrinology*, 32, 627–635. Copyright (2007), with
permission from Elsevier.

Discussion and conclusion

The data presented here extends previous research by demonstrating protective
effects of a high level of physical activity (elite athletes) compared to low levels of
physical activity (untrained men) on both physiological and psychological reactivity to a psychosocial stressor with a task with a social-evaluative character that has
been consistently shown to reliably induce strong stress hormonal responses. Specifically, elite athletes showed reduced salivary free cortisol and heart rate responses,
more calmness, better mood and lower anxiety to the psychosocial stressor.

The finding of markedly lower cortisol responsiveness following psychosocial
stress in trained men compared to untrained men is inconsistent with two previous studies that failed to find significant differences in cortisol responses to a
psychological stressor (Sinyor *et al.*, 1983; Moyna *et al.*, 1999). A possible explanation for the observed differences might lie in the stress protocols, since the
HPA axis is not particularly sensitive to stressor involving cognitive performance like mental arithmetic (Sinyor *et al.*, 1983), as recently shown (Biondi and
Picardi, 1999) compared to a strong reactivity to a psychosocial stressor, which
was employed in this study (Dickerson and Kemeny, 2004). Another possible
explanation lies in the fact that these studies did not include elite sportsmen, but
less highly trained men in their studies. Possibly an alteration of cortisol responsiveness only becomes evident in elite sportsmen.

The finding of lower cardiovascular reactivity to the TSST in elite athletes
is consistent with previous findings on reduced heart rate responsiveness to

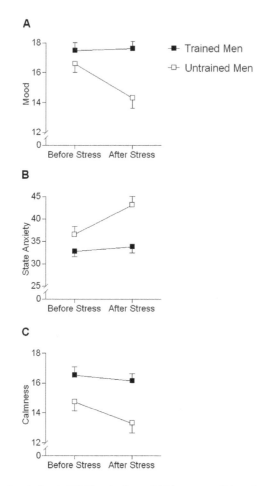

Figure 8.3 Mean levels (with SEM bars) of mood (A), anxiety (B) and calmness (C) before
and after psychosocial stress exposure in trained and untrained men. Reprinted from
Rimmele *et al.* (2007). Trained men show lower cortisol, heart rate and psychological responses to psychosocial stress compared with untrained men. *Psychoneuroendocrinology*, 32, 627–635. Copyright (2007), with permission from Elsevier.

psychological stressors in trained men (Holmes and Roth, 1985; Crews and
Landers, 1987; Moya-Albiol *et al.*, 2001; Spalding *et al.*, 2004). In addition, our
findings are in line with longitudinal studies, which reported that aerobic training leads to lower cardiovascular reactivity to psychological stressors (Throne *et
al.*, 2000; Spalding *et al.*, 2004). Conversely, a recent meta-regression analysis
showed physical fitness to be related to slightly higher cardiovascular reactivity to
psychological stressors (Jackson and Dishman, 2006). The exclusion of elite athletes in the meta-regression analysis may be a reason (albeit not comprehensive)
for this contradictory finding.

With regard to the psychological stress response, the present data build on previous research by demonstrating affective advantages in trained men compared with untrained men. Our finding of better mood in elite athletes throughout the stress protocol is in accordance with previous research showing that acute and chronic exercise improve mood (Netz *et al.*, 2005). Our findings on stress-related anxiety levels are consistent with the results of previous studies, which reported state anxiety to be lower in trained subjects compared to untrained subjects after cessation of stress (Sinyor *et al.*, 1983). As trained men showed lower state anxiety before the stressor as well as a statistical trend toward lower trait anxiety in our study, one may speculate that physically trained subjects generally appraise acute psychosocial stressors as less threatening and more controllable than untrained individuals, which may in turn modulate the activity of the HPA axis and the autonomic nervous system (ANS). For example, longitudinal studies demonstrated a decrease in anxiety following a 12-month or 16-week-long exercise intervention (King *et al.*, 1993; Throne *et al.*, 2000). However, these studies did not examine stress reactivity; they were looking at the relationship between physical activity and anxiety.

The reduced stress reactivity of trained men in our study might be explained by an exercise-induced modulation in stress-responsive hormonal and autonomic nervous systems. Notably, chronic exposure to physical stressors affords redundant activation of the HPA axis and the sympathetic nervous system (Luger *et al.*, 1988; Filaire *et al.*, 2002). Exercise-trained individuals show a reduction in pituitary–adrenocortical activation (Luger *et al.*, 1987; Sothmann *et al.*, 1996) and a lower degree of sympathetic system activation in response to a given absolute workload of physical stress compared to untrained men (Deuster *et al.*, 1989). It is possible that exercise-induced adaptations may also mitigate the responsiveness to other stressors, such as psychosocial stressors. Evidence hinting at this possibility may be drawn from studies that investigate stress reactivity in trained men with different degrees of physical activity. For example, elite athletes have been shown to have lower heart rate reactivity to a psychological stressor than amateur athletes (Moya-Albiol *et al.*, 2001). However, little is known about a potential dose-dependency of physical activity on the moderation of stress responsiveness. In the second study presented here, we therefore set out to test whether different levels of physical activity are associated with different adrenal, cardiovascular and psychological responses to psychosocial stress.

In addition, the favourable effect of physical activity on psychosocial stress may be due to physiological or psychological mechanisms. It is possible that physical activity levels and personality traits or cognitive strategies may interact in moderating the responsiveness to psychosocial stress. For example, personality traits and coping strategies may influence reactivity to psychological stressors (Harrison *et al.*, 2001; Gaab *et al.*, 2005). Athletes have been found to exhibit different characteristics in personality traits (e.g. competitiveness), which in turn have been found to influence stress reactivity (Jones and Swain, 1992; Houston *et al.*, 1997; Frederick, 2000). Hence the second study also set out to assess whether not only different levels in physical activity, but also personality differences moderate reactivity to psychosocial stress.

Physical activity, but not psychological parameters, affects reactivity to psychosocial stress

The findings of the first study showed that elite athletes exhibit lower stress reactivity compared to untrained men. Based on these findings, a second study was conducted to determine potential factors that may explain the lower stress reactivity in elite athletes compared to untrained men. The first question of interest was to assess whether various physical activity levels differentially influence psychosocial stress reactivity. Thus, we included individuals of different physical activity levels (i.e. elite athletes, amateur athletes and untrained men). The second question of interest was whether personality traits and coping strategies, such as competitiveness, which has been shown to be associated with physical activity (Jones and Swain, 1992; Houston *et al.*, 1997; Frederick, 2000), modulate stress reactivity. Several studies have shown that personality traits and coping strategies influence reactivity to psychological stressors (Harrison *et al.*, 2001; Gaab *et al.*, 2005).

Methods

Physical activity and endurance capacity were assessed with a self-report questionnaire and a physical fitness test. The self-report questionnaire asked athletes about the frequency and duration of their participation in exercise activities on a weekly basis and the number of competitions they were involved in per year. The physical fitness test assessed the anaerobic threshold (i.e. the velocity run at a blood lactate concentration of 4 mmol/L), the individual lactate threshold and the maximum running velocity. The physical fitness test was carried out at the end of the sports season in the afternoon. It consisted of a submaximal, non-aversive 4 × 1000 m running test (Held *et al.*, 2000) at self-selected but increasing running speeds (prescribed as slow, medium and fast training speed and maximal velocity) interspersed with short recovery periods of 2 minutes. During recovery, blood samples were taken from the earlobe for assessment of lactate concentration, and perceived exertion was measured with the Borg Scale (Borg *et al.*, 1987).

Based on the physical fitness test and self-report questionnaire, participants were classified into elite athlete or amateur athlete groups. All athletes engaged in ongoing endurance sports activities such as running for a minimum of 3 hours per week. Men were classified as untrained if they were physically inactive and participated for less than one and a half hours per week in any structured exercise.

As in study 1, the Trier Social Stress Test (TSST) was used to induce psychosocial stress (Kirschbaum *et al.*, 1993). Adrenocortical and autonomic responses to psychosocial stress were assessed by repeated measures of salivary free cortisol levels and heart rate. Psychological responses before and after stress exposure were repeatedly assessed with two questionnaires: the state scale of the STAI (Spielberger *et al.*, 1970) measured state anxiety responses to the stressor, and the Multidimensional Mood Questionnaire (Steyer *et al.*, 1997) assessed mood and calmness. General competitiveness was assessed with the Competitiveness Index

(Houston *et al.*, 1992) and sports-specific competitiveness was assessed with the Sports Orientation Questionnaire (SOQ; Gill and Deeter, 1988).

Results

The psychosocial stress protocol induced significant increases in salivary free cortisol levels (Figure 8.4) in all groups of participants. All groups did not differ in their cortisol levels at baseline. Crucially, elite athletes exhibited the lowest cortisol responses compared to the groups of amateur athletes and untrained men. Amateur athletes and untrained men did not differ in their cortisol increases. The stress protocol also induced significant increases in heart rate in all groups (Figure 8.5). Thus there was a significant attenuating effect of physical activity on heart rate, with the lowest heart rate increases during the stress protocol in elite athletes and amateur athletes compared to untrained men.

Considering the psychological variables, state anxiety significantly increased during the anticipation period of the stress protocol in all groups. No significant baseline differences were observed among groups in anxiety, mood and calmness. Interestingly, untrained men showed the highest anxiety levels and elite athletes the lowest anxiety levels throughout the experimental session. The stress protocol also significantly worsened mood and calmness in all groups, with the

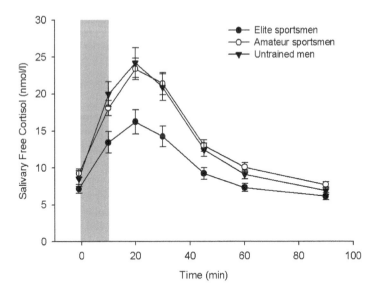

Figure 8.4 Mean salivary free cortisol levels before, during (shaded area) and after a standardized psychosocial stressor (Trier Social Stress Test) in elite athletes, amateur athletes and untrained men. Error bars are standard errors of the mean (SEM). Reprinted from Rimmele et al. (2009). The level of physical activity affects adrenal and cardiovascular reactivity to psychosocial stress. *Psychoneuroendocrinology*, 34, 190–198. Copyright (2009), with permission from Elsevier.

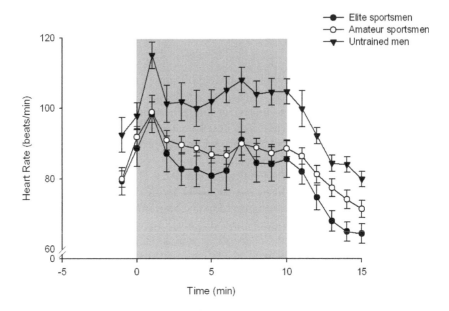

Figure 8.5 Mean heart rates before, during (shaded area) and after a standardized psychosocial stressor in elite athletes, amateur athletes and untrained men. Error bars are SEM. Reprinted from Rimmele *et al.* (2009). The level of physical activity affects adrenal and cardiovascular reactivity to psychosocial stress. *Psychoneuroendocrinology*, 34, 190–198. Copyright (2009), with permission from Elsevier.

lowest mood and calmness scores occurring when subjects were anticipating the stressor.

The groups differed significantly in competitiveness scores as assessed by the Competitiveness Index and the Sports Orientation Questionnaire (SOQ). For the Competitiveness Index, elite athletes showed a higher level of competitiveness than amateur athletes and untrained men. For the SOQ, elite athletes displayed the highest competitiveness, with amateur athletes showing intermediate, and untrained men the lowest competitiveness levels. In order to determine whether differences in competitiveness among groups may modulate stress responses, a moderator analysis was conducted (Baron and Kenny, 1986). However, competitiveness did not moderate group differences in cortisol, heart rate and psychological responses to stress.

Discussion

In the present study, we examined whether different levels of physical activity are associated with different psychological, adrenal and autonomic responses to a standardized psychosocial stressor. In addition, we tested the potential influence of competitiveness on the relationship between physical activity and stress reactivity. As in the previous study, the stress protocol significantly increased cortisol and heart rate responses, worsened mood and calmness, and increased state anxiety in all groups. More importantly, the data of this study suggest that different levels of physical activity differentially affect the physiological and psychological reactivity to psychosocial stress. As such, the group with the highest physical activity level (elite athletes) showed the lowest stress reactivity in all assessed parameters (i.e. in cortisol, heart rate and state anxiety). Interestingly, the reactivity of the sympathetic nervous system to stress was revealed to be sensitive to higher levels of physical activity (elite and amateur athletes), whereas cortisol responses were attenuated only in elite athletes, but not in amateur athletes. The observed differences in competitiveness between the groups were not associated with differences in stress reactivity.

Our finding of lower cortisol responses to psychosocial stress in elite athletes compared with untrained men is consistent with the findings of the study presented above in another sample of elite athletes and untrained men (Rimmele et al., 2007). The similar cortisol responses in amateur athletes and untrained men observed here are also consistent with previous studies that likewise did not reveal differences in cortisol reactivity to psychological stressors among amateur athletes of differing levels of fitness or between amateur athletes and sedentary subjects (Sinyor et al., 1983; Moyna et al., 1999).

Both elite athletes and amateur athletes showed significantly lower heart rate responses to stress compared with untrained men, replicating previous reports from several cross-sectional studies (Heidbreder et al., 1983; Holmes and Roth, 1985; Brooke and Long, 1987; Claytor, 1991; Rimmele et al., 2007). In addition, a longitudinal study showed that aerobic training reduces the cardiovascular response to psychological stress (Spalding et al., 2004). In contrast, a recent meta-regression analysis reported cardiorespiratory fitness to be linked to slightly stronger cardiovascular responses to psychological stress (Jackson and Dishman, 2006). Different types of psychological stressors, the exclusion of elite athletes, differences in physical activity and fitness levels, variations in age and gender of the subjects, the method of measurement, and the time of day of stress induction of the studies included in the meta-regression analysis may be reasons explaining this divergent outcome.

It is important to note that the comparison of physiological changes across the three groups revealed a dissociation of 'dose gradients' of physical activity between sympathetic nervous system (heart rate) and HPA axis (cortisol) responses. Only elite athletes showed consistently lower stress responses compared with untrained men both in heart rate and cortisol responses to the psychosocial stressor, whereas amateur athletes showed lower heart rate but similar cortisol responses as compared to untrained men. Although the mechanisms underlying this dissociation are unknown, it might be suggested that the sympathetic nervous system (as the main regulator of heart rate) is more sensitive to the adaptive consequences of physical activity and that potential adaptations of the HPA axis occur later on, at a higher level of physical activity. Chronic physical exercise is associated with reduced HPA axis activation if the experimental stressor is of the same absolute physical intensity (Luger *et al.*, 1987), and cortisol reactivity to a physical stressor has been found to correlate with the reactivity to a psychological stressor (Singh *et al.*, 1999). In this context, it is possible that only a markedly enhanced level of physical activity, such as in elite athletes, rather than graded increases causes a significant adaptation of the HPA response that may generalize to other stressors.

With regard to the psychological stress response, elite athletes showed the lowest, amateur athletes intermediate and untrained men the highest state anxiety responses, which is in agreement with previous findings (Sinyor *et al.*, 1983; Rimmele *et al.*, 2007). Acute periods of exercise as well as prolonged exposure (over 10 weeks) to aerobic exercise are related to a reduction in anxiety (Petruzzello *et al.*, 1997; Salmon, 2001). A linear 'dose-dependent' relationship between exercise and affective psychological adaptations, such as anxiety, has been proposed (Petruzzello *et al.*, 1997). Our findings suggest that this dose–response relationship may translate into changes in state anxiety to a psychosocial stressor. However, whether the dose–response relationship is linear cannot be determined from our findings.

We also examined whether competitiveness moderates psychosocial stress reactivity. Both general and sports-specific competitiveness levels were highest in elite athletes, differing markedly from levels in amateur athletes or untrained men, which concurs with many previous reports (Houston *et al.*, 1997). However, competitiveness did not moderate adrenal and autonomic stress responsiveness. Thus, higher competitiveness may be linked to a higher level of physical activity, but seems to be unrelated to stress reactivity.

Summary and outlook

Employing a cross-stressor adaptation hypothesis, several researchers have argued that the adaptation of stress systems as a result of physical activity may influence physiological stress reactivity to physical stress, and also to non-exercise stress, such as psychological stress (de Geus *et al.*, 1990; Sothmann *et al.*, 1996). However, the extent to which physical activity may reduce the responsiveness to psychological stress, and may act as a stress-protective factor, thus preventing stress-related disorders, is still a debated issue. Cross-sectional, as well as longitudinal studies, which sought to determine the influence of physical activity on stress reactivity to mental, psychological stressors yielded inconsistent findings (Claytor, 1991; Cox, 1991; Sothmann *et al.*, 1991; Sothmann *et al.*, 1996).

The first study reported here was aimed at resolving some of the inconsistencies found using an extreme group approach, the Trier Social Stress Test, a naturalistic highly potent stressor, and broad measurements of psychological and physiological stress reactivity. The goal of the second study was to further elucidate the potential dose-dependency of physical activity on psychosocial stress reactivity and the influence of other factors shown to play a role in stress responsiveness, such as personality traits like competitiveness. Using this approach the influence of three different levels of physical activity on psychological stress reactivity was investigated: elite athletes, amateur athletes and untrained men.

In both studies, elite athletes exhibited significantly reduced heart rate, cortisol and state anxiety responses to the psychosocial stressor compared to untrained men. The second study additionally revealed a dose-dependency of physical activity levels on psychosocial stress reactivity. While elite athletes showed the lowest cardiovascular reactivity, the lowest cortisol levels and the lowest state anxiety responses compared to both amateur athletes and untrained men, amateur athletes showed, like elite athletes, lower responses in cardiovascular and psychological parameters compared to untrained men. However, in contrast to elite athletes, amateur athletes showed the same degree of cortisol responses to psychosocial stressors as untrained men.

The presented results thus do not show a simple dose–gradient relation of physical activity on psychological stress reactivity. The mechanisms underlying the difference in reactivity of the SNS and the HPA axis in amateur athletes compared to elite athletes are yet to be elucidated. On a physiological level, exercise induces changes in SNS reactivity to stress as well as in the HPA axis. These exercise-induced adaptations to physical stress may lead to a better adaptation of the organism and more efficient physiological functioning under exposure to psychological stress (Sothmann *et al.*, 1996). The lower heart rate reactivity of both amateur and elite athletes in our study may be explained by an exercise-induced adaptation of the cardiovascular system. Acute aerobic exercise is characterized by cardiac–vagal withdrawal and beta-adrenergic activation, leading to a rise in heart rate (Moya-Albiol *et al.*, 2001). Chronic aerobic exercise can mitigate the chronotropic heart response to sympathetic activation, while increasing its ionotropic response (Goldberg *et al.*, 1996; Jackson and Dishman, 2006).

Furthermore, chronic aerobic exercise can lead to a decrease in cardiac-sympathetic drive (Hopkins *et al.*, 1996; Spina *et al.*, 1998). These exercise-induced adaptations may explain the lower heart rate reactivity in trained as compared to untrained men not only for physical but also for psychological stress as found in the above-described and previous studies (Dishman, 1997; Dishman *et al.*, 2006; Rimmele *et al.*, 2007, 2009). In sum, the lower heart rate in trained subjects speaks for the moderating role of physical training for reactions of the SNS to psychological stress. This is in line with the cross-stressor adaptation hypothesis (O'Sullivan and Bell, 2000; Krieger *et al.*, 2001). In addition, chronic exposure to physical stress leads to repeated activation of the HPA axis (Sothmann *et al.*, 1996).

It has been suggested that the repeated activation leads to a habituation of the HPA hormonal response to exercise (Luger *et al.*, 1988; Filaire *et al.*, 2002). Specifically, exercise-trained men show a reduction in HPA activation in response to physical stress (Sothmann *et al.*, 1996; Gaab *et al.*, 2005). Interestingly this reduction in HPA activation is lower for elite athletes than for amateur athletes (Luger *et al.*, 1987). The divergent findings of the second study may thus be ascribed to differences in exercise-induced adaptations between the HPA axis and the SNS. Possibly, the SNS adapts faster than the HPA axis to repeated physical stress. This may translate to a better adaptation of the SNS but not the HPA axis to psychosocial stress as observed for amateur athletes.

In contrast, when you have a physical activity level that is as high as in the investigated elite athletes, an adaptation of both the SNS and HPA axis to physical stress may translate to lower reactivity of both the SNS and HPA axis to psychosocial stress, as observed for the elite athletes in the presented studies.

Consistent with physiological stress responses, athletes showed significantly lower psychological stress reactivity than untrained men in both studies. This finding is consistent with a previous study reporting state anxiety to be lower in trained subjects compared to untrained subjects after the cessation of stress (Kudielka *et al.*, 2004). In addition, in the second study, state anxiety varied with the degree of physical activity: elite athletes showed the lowest, amateur athletes intermediate and untrained men the highest state anxiety responses, which is in agreement with previous findings (Sinyor *et al.*, 1983; Rimmele *et al.*, 2007). Intervention studies have shown that acute periods of exercise as well as prolonged exposure (over 10 weeks) to aerobic exercise reduces trait anxiety (Sinyor *et al.*, 1983; Petruzzello *et al.*, 1997; Salmon, 2001). These exercise-modulated lower trait anxiety levels in trained men may in turn lead to lower state anxiety responses to a stress situation in trained vs. untrained men. Future studies should investigate whether there is indeed a linear 'dose-dependent' relationship between exercise and affective psychological adaptations (Petruzzello *et al.*, 1997), such as anxiety responses to a psychosocial stressor.

Overall, the presented results suggest that physical activity is associated with a decrease in adrenal, autonomic and psychological responses to psychosocial stress. These findings could inform the development of preventive measures against psychiatric and cardiovascular diseases. Psychiatric disorders have been associated with dysregulation of the HPA axis (Crews and Landers, 1987; Jackson and Dishman, 2006), which is activated during stress. It has been proposed that exaggerated cardiovascular reactions to psychological stress contribute to the pathogenesis of cardiovascular disease (Ehlert and Straub, 1998; Ehlert *et al.*, 2001). As the presented studies show that physical activity is associated with decreased psychosocial stress reactivity, it is possible that physical activity prevents exaggerated stress reactivity and therefore could help prevent the development of psychiatric or cardiovascular diseases. A better understanding of the underlying mechanisms of physical activity on stress-responsive physiological systems could help in the development of multidimensional stress prevention programmes (e.g. combining physical activity components with mental training strategies).

Limitations of the present studies

While in both presented studies a cross-sectional study design was used, the data presented here does not allow a causal interpretation of the effects of physical activity on stress responsiveness. Prospective longitudinal studies are needed in order to confirm that physical activity decreases stress responses and, as a long-term effect, may protect against stress-related disorders. Similarly, the relationship of the type and the amount of physical activity and the possible influence of psychological variables in terms of stress protection should also be investigated in longitudinal study designs. While our participants were selected to be medium- to long-distance runners, our study is limited in that we did not assess complete data on the other kinds of physical activity that they were carrying out. As our total sample included healthy young men, the results cannot be generalized to the population as a whole, and particularly not to persons of older age than the participants in our studies.

Also, aside from the physiological and psychological make-up of participants, underlying genetic mechanisms could be investigated, as physical fitness is partially determined genetically.

Lastly, the neurobiological mechanisms underlying the interplay between physical activity and psychosocial stress reactivity should be investigated in order to better understand the stress protective mechanisms of physical activity. Findings from animal studies, together with new findings in human studies that show how exercise affects the human brain (e.g. Erickson *et al.*, 2011), could lay a foundation for the development of brain imaging and pharmacological studies in order to investigate the stress protective neurobiological underpinnings of exercise in humans.

References

Babyak, M., Blumenthal, J. A., Herman, S., et al. (2000). Exercise treatment for major depression: maintenance of therapeutic benefit at 10 months. *Psychosomatic Medicine*, 62, 633–638.

Baron, R.M. and Kenny, D.A. (1986). The moderator-mediator variable distinction in social psychological research: conceptual, strategic, and statistical considerations. *Journal of Personality and Social Psychology*, 51, 1173-1182.

Biondi, M. and Picardi, A. (1999). Psychological stress and neuroendocrine function in humans: the last two decades of research. *Psychotherapy and Psychosomatics*, 68, 114–150.

Borg, G., Hassmen, P. and Lagerstrom, M. (1987). Perceived exertion related to heart rate and blood lactate during arm and leg exercise. *European Journal of Applied Physiology and Occupational Physiology*, 56, 679–685.

Boutcher, S. H. and Landers, D. M. (1988). The effects of vigorous exercise on anxiety, heart rate, and alpha activity of runners and nonrunners. *Psychophysiology*, 25, 696–702.

Brooke, S. T. and Long, B. C. (1987). Efficiency of coping with a real-life stressor: a multimodal comparison of aerobic fitness. *Psychophysiology*, 24, 173–180.

Cacioppo, J. T., Berntson, G. G., Malarkey, W. B., et al. (1998). Autonomic, neuroendocrine, and immune responses to psychological stress: the reactivity hypothesis. *Annals of the New York Academy of Sciences*, 840, 664–673.

Claytor, R. P. (1991). Stress reactivity: hemodynamic adjustments in trained and untrained humans. *Medicine and Science in Sports and Exercise*, 23, 873–881.

Claytor, R. P., Cox, R. H., Howley, E. T., Lawler, K. A. and Lawler, J. E. (1988). Aerobic power and cardiovascular response to stress. *Journal of Applied Physiology*, 65, 1416–1423.

Cohen, S., Kamarck, T. and Mermelstein, R. (1983). A global measure of perceived stress. *Journal of Health and Social Behavior*, 24, 385–396.

Cox, R. H. (1991). Exercise training and response to stress: insights from an animal model. *Medicine and Science in Sports and Exercise*, 23, 853–859.

Crews, D. J. and Landers, D. M. (1987). A meta-analytic review of aerobic fitness and reactivity to psychosocial stressors. *Medicine and Science in Sports and Exercise*, 19, S114–120.

de Geus, E. J. and van Doornen, L. J. (1993). The effects of fitness training on the physiological stress response. *Work and Stress*, 7, 141–159.

de Geus, E. J., van Doornen, L. J., de Visser, D. C. and Orlebeke, J. F. (1990). Existing and training induced differences in aerobic fitness: their relationship to physiological response patterns during different types of stress. *Psychophysiology*, 27, 457–478.

de Geus, E. J., van Doornen, L. J. and Orlebeke, J. F. (1993). Regular exercise and aerobic fitness in relation to psychological make-up and physiological stress reactivity. *Psychosomatic Medicine*, 55, 347–363.

Deuster, P. A., Chrousos, G. P., Luger, A., *et al.* (1989). Hormonal and metabolic responses of untrained, moderately trained, and highly trained men to three exercise intensities. *Metabolism*, 38, 141–148.

Dickerson, S. S. and Kemeny, M. E. (2004). Acute stressors and cortisol responses: a theoretical integration and synthesis of laboratory research. *Psychological Bulletin*, 130, 355–391.

Dishman, R. K. (1997). Brain monoamines, exercise, and behavioral stress: animal models. *Medicine and Science in Sports and Exercise*, 29, 63–74.

Dishman, R. K., Berthoud, H. R., Booth, F. W., *et al.* (2006). Neurobiology of exercise. *Obesity*, 14, 345–356.

Ehlert, U. and Straub, R. (1998). Physiological and emotional response to psychological stressors in psychiatric and psychosomatic disorders. *Annals of the New York Academy of Sciences*, 851, 477–486.

Ehlert, U., Gaab, J. and Heinrichs, M. (2001). Psychoneuroendocrinological contributions to the etiology of depression, posttraumatic stress disorder, and stress-related bodily disorders: the role of the hypothalamus-pituitary-adrenal axis. *Biological Psychology*, 57, 141–152.

Erickson, K. I., Voss, M. W., Prakash, R. S., *et al.* (2011). Exercise training increases size of hippocampus and improves memory. *Proceedings of the National Academy of Sciences USA*, 108, 3017–3022.

Filaire, E., Legrand, B., Bret, K., Sagnol, M., Cottet-Emard, J. M. and Pequignot, J. M. (2002). Psychobiologic responses to 4 days of increased training and recovery in cyclists. *International Journal of Sports Medicine*, 23, 588–594.

Frederick, C. M. (2000). Competitiveness: relations with GPA, locus of control, sex, and athletic status. *Perceptual and Motor Skills*, 90, 413–414.

Gaab, J., Rohleder, N., Nater, U. M. and Ehlert, U. (2005). Psychological determinants of the cortisol stress response: the role of anticipatory cognitive appraisal. *Psychoneuroendocrinology*, 30, 599–610.

Gill, D. L. and Deeter, T. E. (1988). Development of the Sports Orientation Questionnaire. *Research Quaterly for Exercise and Sports*, 59, 191–202.

Gold, P. W., Goodwin, F. K. and Chrousos, G. P. (1988). Clinical and biochemical manifestations of depression. Relation to the neurobiology of stress (2). *New England Journal of Medicine*, 319, 413–420.

Goldberg, A. D., Becker, L. C., Bonsall, R., *et al.* (1996). Ischemic, hemodynamic, and neurohormonal responses to mental and exercise stress. Experience from the Psychophysiological Investigations of Myocardial Ischemia Study (PIMI). *Circulation*, 94, 2402–2409.

Harrison, L. K., Denning, S., Easton, H. L., *et al.* (2001). The effects of competition and competitiveness on cardiovascular activity. *Psychophysiology*, 38, 601–606.

Heidbreder, E., Ziegler, A., Heidland, A. and Kirsten, R. (1983). [Mental stress and sports. Does physical activity increase stress tolerance?]. *Die Medizinische Welt*, 34, 43–47.

Heinrichs, M., Meinlschmidt, G., Neumann, I., *et al.* (2001). Effects of suckling on hypothalamic-pituitary-adrenal axis responses to psychosocial stress in postpartum lactating women. *Journal of Clinical Endocrinology and Metabolism*, 86, 4798–4804.

Held, T., Steiner, R., Huebner, K., Tschopp, M., Peltola, K. and Marti, B. (2000). Self-selected submaxial running velocities as predictors of endurance capacity. *Schweizerische Zeitschrift für Sportmedizin und Sporttraumatologie*, 48, 64–68.

Holmes, D. S. and Roth, D. L. (1985). Association of aerobic fitness with pulse rate and subjective responses to psychological stress. *Psychophysiology*, 22, 525–529.

Hopkins, M. G., Spina, R. J. and Ehsani, A. A. (1996). Enhanced beta-adrenergic-mediated cardiovascular responses in endurance athletes. *Journal of Applied Physiology*, 80, 516–521.

Houston, J. M., Carter, D. and Smither, R. D. (1997). Competitiveness in elite professional athletes. *Perceptual and Motor Skills*, 84, 1447–1457.

Houston, J. M., Farese, D. M. and La Du, T. J. (1992). Assessing competitiveness: a validation study of the Competitiveness Index. *Personality and Individual Differences*, 13, 1153–1156.

Hull, E. M., Young, S. H. and Ziegler, M. G. (1984). Aerobic fitness affects cardiovascular and catecholamine responses to stressors. *Psychophysiology*, 21, 353–360.

Jackson, E. M. and Dishman, R. K. (2006). Cardiorespiratory fitness and laboratory stress: a meta-regression analysis. *Psychophysiology*, 43, 57–72.

Jones, G. and Swain, A. (1992). Intensity and direction as dimensions of competitive state anxiety and relationships with competitiveness. *Perceptual and Motor Skills*, 74, 467–472.

Kalia, M. (2002). Assessing the economic impact of stress – the modern day hidden epidemic. *Metabolism*, 51, 49–53.

Ketelhut, R. G., Franz, I. W. and Scholze, J. (2004). Regular exercise as an effective approach in antihypertensive therapy. *Medicine and Science in Sports and Exercise*, 36, 4–8.

King, A. C., Taylor, C. B. and Haskell, W. L. (1993). Effects of differing intensities and formats of 12 months of exercise training on psychological outcomes in older adults. *Health Psychology*, 12, 292–300.

Kirschbaum, C. and Hellhammer, D. H. (1989). Salivary cortisol in psychobiological research: an overview. *Neuropsychobiology*, 22, 150–169.

Kirschbaum, C. and Hellhammer, D. H. (1994). Salivary cortisol in psychoneuroendocrine research: recent developments and applications. *Psychoneuroendocrinology*, 19, 313–333.

Kirschbaum, C., Pirke, K. M. and Hellhammer, D. H. (1993). The 'Trier Social Stress Test' – a tool for investigating psychobiological stress responses in a laboratory setting. *Neuropsychobiology*, 28, 76–81.

Kirschbaum, C., Kudielka, B. M., Gaab, J., Schommer, N. C. and Hellhammer, D. H. (1999). Impact of gender, menstrual cycle phase, and oral contraceptives on the activity of the hypothalamus-pituitary-adrenal axis. *Psychosomatic Medicine*, 61, 154–162.

Krieger, E. M., Da Silva, G. J. and Negrao, C. E. (2001). Effects of exercise training on baroreflex control of the cardiovascular system. *Annals of the New York Academy of Sciences*, 940, 338–347.

Kudielka, B. M., Buske-Kirschbaum, A., Hellhammer, D. H. and Kirschbaum, C. (2004). HPA axis responses to laboratory psychosocial stress in healthy elderly adults, younger adults, and children: impact of age and gender. *Psychoneuroendocrinology*, 29, 83–98.

Luger, A., Deuster, P. A., Kyle, S. B., *et al.* (1987). Acute hypothalamic-pituitary-adrenal responses to the stress of treadmill exercise. Physiologic adaptations to physical training. *New England Journal of Medicine*, 316, 1309–1315.

Luger, A., Deuster, P. A., Gold, P. W., Loriaux, D. L. and Chrousos, G. P. (1988). Hormonal responses to the stress of exercise. *Advances in Experimental Medicine and Biology*, 245, 273–280.

McEwen, B. S. (1998). Protective and damaging effects of stress mediators. *New England Journal of Medicine*, 338, 171–179.

McEwen, B. S. (2000). The neurobiology of stress: from serendipity to clinical relevance. *Brain Research*, 886, 172–189.

McEwen, B. S. (2002). Protective and damaging effects of stress mediators: the good and bad sides of the response to stress. *Metabolism*, 51, 2–4.

Motl, R. W., Birnbaum, A. S., Kubik, M. Y. and Dishman, R. K. (2004). Naturally occurring changes in physical activity are inversely related to depressive symptoms during early adolescence. *Psychosomatic Medicine*, 66, 336–342.

Moya-Albiol, L., Salvador, A., Costa, R., *et al.* (2001). Psychophysiological responses to the Stroop Task after a maximal cycle ergometry in elite sportsmen and physically active subjects. *International Journal of Psychophysiology*, 40, 47–59.

Moyna, N. M., Bodnar, J. D., Goldberg, H. R., Shurin, M. S., Robertson, R. J. and Rabin, B. S. (1999). Relation between aerobic fitness level and stress induced alterations in neuroendocrine and immune function. *International Journal of Sports Medicine*, 20, 136–141.

Netz, Y., Wu, M. J., Becker, B. J. and Tenenbaum, G. (2005). Physical activity and psychological well-being in advanced age: a meta-analysis of intervention studies. *Psychology and Aging*, 20, 272–284.

O'Sullivan, S. E. and Bell, C. (2000). The effects of exercise and training on human cardiovascular reflex control. *Journal of the Autonomic Nervous System*, 81, 16–24.

Petruzzello, S. J., Jones, A. C. and Tate, A. K. (1997). Affective responses to acute exercise: a test of opponent-process theory. *Journal of Sports Medicine and Physical Fitness*, 37, 205–212.

Rimmele, U., Zellweger, B. C., Marti, B., *et al.* (2007). Trained men show lower cortisol, heart rate and psychological responses to psychosocial stress compared with untrained men. *Psychoneuroendocrinology*, 32, 627–635.

Rimmele, U., Seiler, R., Marti, B., Wirtz, P. H., Ehlert, U. and Heinrichs, M. (2009). The level of physical activity affects adrenal and cardiovascular reactivity to psychosocial stress. *Psychoneuroendocrinology*, 34, 190–198.

Salmon, P. (2001). Effects of physical exercise on anxiety, depression, and sensitivity to stress: a unifying theory. *Clinical Psychology Review*, 21, 33–61.

Selye, H. (1950). Stress and the general adaptation syndrome. *British Medical Journal*, 4667, 1383–1392.

Senkfor, A. J. and Williams, J. M. (1995). The moderating effects of aerobic fitness and mental training on stress reactivity. *Journal of Sport Behavior*, 18, 130–156.

Singh, A., Petrides, J. S., Gold, P. W., Chrousos, G. P. and Deuster, P. A. (1999). Differential hypothalamic-pituitary-adrenal axis reactivity to psychological and physical stress. *Journal of Clinical Endocrinology and Metabolism*, 84, 1944–1948.

Sinyor, D., Schwartz, S. G., Peronnet, F., Brisson, G. and Seraganian, P. (1983). Aerobic fitness level and reactivity to psychosocial stress: physiological, biochemical, and subjective measures. *Psychosomatic Medicine*, 45, 205–217.

Sinyor, D., Golden, M., Steinert, Y. and Seraganian, P. (1986). Experimental manipulation of aerobic fitness and the response to psychosocial stress: heart rate and self-report measures. *Psychosomatic Medicine*, 48, 324–337.

Sothmann, M. S., Hart, B. A. and Horn, T. S. (1991). Plasma catecholamine response to acute psychological stress in humans: relation to aerobic fitness and exercise training. *Medicine and Science in Sports and Exercise*, 23, 860–867.

Sothmann, M. S., Buckworth, J., Claytor, R. P., Cox, R. H., White-Welkley, J. E. and Dishman, R. K. (1996). Exercise training and the cross-stressor adaptation hypothesis. *Exercise and Sport Sciences Reviews*, 24, 267–287.

Spalding, T. W., Lyon, L. A., Steel, D. H. and Hatfield, B. D. (2004). Aerobic exercise training and cardiovascular reactivity to psychological stress in sedentary young normotensive men and women. *Psychophysiology*, 41, 552–562.

Spielberger, C. D., Gorsuch, R. L. and Lushene, R. E. (1970). *Manual for the State-Trait Anxiety Inventory*. Palo Alto, CA: Consult. Psychologists Press.

Spina, R. J., Turner, M. J. and Ehsani, A. A. (1998). Beta-adrenergic-mediated improvement in left ventricular function by exercise training in older men. *American Journal of Physiology*, 274, H397–404.

Steptoe, A. (1991). Invited review. The links between stress and illness. *Journal of Psychosomatic Research*, 35, 633–644.

Steptoe, A., Moses, J., Mathews, A. and Edwards, S. (1990). Aerobic fitness, physical activity, and psychophysiological reactions to mental tasks. *Psychophysiology*, 27, 264–274.

Steptoe, A., Kearsley, N. and Walters, N. (1993). Cardiovascular activity during mental stress following vigorous exercise in sportsmen and inactive men. *Psychophysiology*, 30, 245–252.

Steyer, R., Schwenkmezger, P., Notz, P. and Eid, M. (1997). *Der Mehrdimensionale Befindlichkeitsbogen (MDBF) [Multidimensional Mood Questionnaire]*. Hogrefe, Göttingen.

Talbot, L. A., Morrell, C. H., Metter, E. J. and Fleg, J. L. (2002). Comparison of cardiorespiratory fitness versus leisure time physical activity as predictors of coronary events in men aged < or = 65 years and > 65 years. *American Journal of Cardiology*, 89, 1187–1192.

Throne, L. C., Bartholomew, J. B., Craig, J. and Farrar, R. P. (2000). Stress reactivity in fire fighters: an exercise intervention. *International Journal of Stress Management*, 7, 235–246.

Tsigos, C. and Chrousos, G. P. (2002). Hypothalamic-pituitary-adrenal axis, neuroendocrine factors and stress. *Journal of Psychosomatic Research*, 53, 865–871.

Vanitallie, T. B. (2002). Stress: a risk factor for serious illness. *Metabolism*, 51, 40–45.

Vining, R. F., McGinley, R. A., Maksvytis, J. J. and Ho, K. Y. (1983). Salivary cortisol: a better measure of adrenal cortical function than serum cortisol. *Annals of Clinical Biochemistry*, 20 (Pt 6), 329–335.

9 Spectators' physiological responses to sport events

Silvan Steiner

Considerable research has been carried out to investigate athletes' physiological reactions to sport performances. Previous chapters have offered insight and given an overview about the progress in this field of research. At the same time, only a few studies have been conducted to understand the effects of sport events on the physiological system of attending spectators. In this chapter we provide a brief outline of the physiological reactions reported as a result of attending sport events. A pilot study of the on-line effects of watching a soccer game on parameters described in earlier chapters of this book is then described and recommendations for future studies given.

Reported influences of sport events on the physiological systems of spectators

As for psychological variables (e.g. Sloan, 1979; Schwarz *et al.*, 1987; Hirt *et al.*, 1992), various studies have been conducted to test for the effects sport events can have on the physiological systems of spectators and attending athletes . Studies investigating the cardiovascular system of sport spectators have shown increased sympathetic activation during sport events. Rose and Dunn (1964) found that the heart rate of American Football viewers were elevated during games. Increases in heart rate were observed throughout the competition but not during games in which the outcome was determined early. Similarly, increased heart rate has been reported for spectators of soccer games (Hüllemann *et al.*, 1970; Hijzen and Slangen, 1985; Harrison *et al.*, 2000).

Epidemiologic research has also been undertaken to test the notion that sport events affect the cardiovascular systems of spectators. Various studies have contributed indirect support for this, revealing increased mortality due to myocardial infarction during phases of championship tournaments (Katz *et al.*, 2005, 2006) or after single games (Witte *et al.*, 2000; Carroll *et al.*, 2002). This has been suggested to be a consequence of sustained sympathetic adrenal–medullary (SAM) system activation caused by stress associated with watching soccer games. However, another study failed to document this effect after soccer games (Brunekreef and Hoek, 2002).

Finally, Berthier and Boulay (2003) reported a decrease in nationwide heart attacks in France after their win in the 1998 World Cup Soccer final over

Brazil. As a consequence, the latter discussed the existence of salutogenic effects of vicarious winning. In sum, epidemiologic research thus has contributed findings that are mixed at best.

Cortisol is a steroid hormone extensively tested for its prominent role in the physiological stress response (see Chapter 3). The hormone is an indicator of the hypothalamic–pituitary–adrenal (HPA) axis and has been reported to increase after exposure to psychological and/or physiological stressors (Dickerson and Kemeny, 2004). Data on the reactions of spectators to sport events in terms of cortisol are not available, but in a study on soccer coaches it was found that the cortisol concentrations increased over 100% from before the games to the half-time breaks and fell again below pre-game levels 1 hour after termination of the games (Kugler *et al.*, 1996). This study measured cortisol responses throughout the game. In contrast, studies on inactive team members attending their team games have reported either decreases or no changes in cortisol from before-game to after-game concentrations for the case of ice hockey (Tegelman *et al.*, 1988) and soccer (Edwards *et al.*, 2006).

In summary, the available literature on cortisol reactions to sport events comes from studies with fairly different measurement techniques. The mentioned results are somewhat inconsistent and the respective studies focus on non-playing team members and coaches rather than spectators. Therefore, from these results it seems problematic to deduce a hypothesis considering the course of cortisol for people who are not physically participating but are spectating. The inclusion of measurements during ongoing games would allow more comparable measurement setups, and help to clarify some of the differences found for coaches and athletes.

Some investigations have been dedicated to the testosterone response to sport events. Testosterone is the final product of the hypothalamic–pituitary–gonadal (HPG) axis (see Chapter 4). While not directly involved in the human physiological stress response, the hormone has been proposed to be sensitive to the scoring of attended games. Bernhardt *et al.* (1998) were the first to report a winner/loser effect in spectators of basketball and soccer games. After completion of highly competitive basketball and soccer games, supporters of the victorious teams showed increases in testosterone, while the hormone decreased in supporters of the losing team. This work was extended by Carré and Putnam (2010) who demonstrated a similar testosterone-stimulating effect after watching oneself win a previous competitive sport interaction.

Another study by Edwards *et al.* (2006) analysed testosterone reactivity in soccer players who played a league match, and compared it to the reactivity of those members of the team who were present but did not play. These reserve players resemble spectators more closely than the participants in the study by Carré and Putnam (2010). For a game won, no statistically significant changes in before-game to after-game testosterone concentrations were found for either players or reserve players. Comparing the changes in testosterone between the two groups, the researchers reported a significant player/reserve effect: the testosterone concentration of the players increased while the concentration of the reserve athletes decreased.

As for cortisol reactions of spectators and attendees at sport events, testosterone reactions to sport events have not yet been the focus of much research. The observance of elevated testosterone concentrations after winning games does not go uncontested and needs further research.

Pilot study on the physiological on-line reactions of spectators to a broadcast soccer game

Overall, our knowledge of the physiological changes accompanying the attendance of sport events is limited. Support for increased activation of the autonomous nervous system (ANS) accompanying sport events can be found. The scarce literature on endocrinological reaction patterns report inconsistent findings. Most studies employing such parameters to track physiological reactions to sport events have only considered measurement points before and after events, and do not describe reactions during the ongoing games. Data on salivary alpha-amylase (sAA, see Chapter 6) and heart rate variability (HRV), another parameter used for inferring activation of the ANS (Task Force of the European Society and Cardiology and the North American Society of Pacing and Electrophysiology, 1996), have not been presented yet. The pilot study by Steiner *et al.* (2011) outlined in the following sections appears to be the first study to examine the sensitivity of these parameters to watching a sport event.

Methods

The physiological reactions of seven healthy males to a live broadcast soccer game were examined in a controlled laboratory setting. Only male participants between 20 and 30 years of age (M = 24.00; SD = 2.7) were included in the study, because both sex and age are known to account for differences in both mean concentration and reactivity of several of the parameters at focus. The subjects were instructed to refrain from consuming alcohol and caffeine for 48 hours, and to refrain from eating 2 hours prior to the investigation. Furthermore, they were advised not to physically exhaust themselves for 24 hours prior to the investigation. Participants arrived 90 minutes before the onset of the game. This time was scheduled to make sure they spent the time before kickoff under comparable conditions in order to establish some sort of a baseline state.

All participants stayed in the same room, where they watched the game on a big screen. Each participant was provided a separate table to sit at and from where to watch the game. They were instructed to stay at their assigned places. The use of the restroom was restricted to the halftime break to make sure that no walking or moving around during the game caused artefacts.

Heart rate, the high- and low-frequency spectrum power of the HRV (HF, LF), sAA, cortisol and testosterone were measured to delineate on-line responses to the broadcast. Several mood variables (e.g. perceived stress and bodily arousal) were included to test for changes during the sport event, and to explore their interplay with physiological variables. The measurement alignments for all physiological and psychological variables incorporated time points before, during, and after the game. The game was scheduled for the evening. This time of day is well suited for studies on cortisol and testosterone because the concentrations of both parameters are reported to be relatively stable at that time, a precondition for the detection of event-related alterations (Dabbs, 1990; Dickerson and Kemeny, 2004).

Results

The game ended in a goalless draw. Data analysis revealed significant changes for heart rate, with peak values during the game. It also revealed sAA to be affected by the game. Highest concentrations were measured during the game time and lowest concentrations after completion of the game. No statistically significant changes were shown for HF, LF, cortisol and testosterone. For the self-report measures, the game had an effect on the perception of bodily arousal, with highest ratings obtained during the game. Also, self-reported stress tended to be higher during the game.

The results showed increased activation of the sympathetic nervous system (SNS) during the soccer game as indicated by the changes in sAA and heart rate. HF power, an index of parasympathetic activity, and LF power, discussed to be influenced by both branches of the ANS did not change throughout the course of the event.

Discussion

To what extent the activation of the SNS might be related to reported increases in heart attacks during phases of championship tournaments is a question to be addressed in future studies. The course of sAA paralleled the chart lines for the perception of bodily arousal and stress, all showing elevated values during the two halves compared to the lower values before the game, in the halftime break, and after the game. Heart rate did not follow that same pattern, but steadily increased to reach highest levels shortly before the final whistle, a replication of the finding by Rose and Dunn (1964). The considerable similarities in the courses of sAA and self-reported stress variables are interesting in the context of identifying an objective biological parameter that is correlated with the subjective perception of stress in a sport competition's atmosphere. At the same time, it could be some support the proposition that sAA is a more sensitive marker for psychological stress than heart rate (van Stegeren *et al.*, 2006).

Although changes in cortisol and testosterone concentrations missed significance, both hormones decreased by trend during the time of observation. For spectators, cortisol concentrations measured in the halftime break were the lowest of all samples taken. This contrasts with the finding of increased cortisol concentrations during the halftime break reported for soccer coaches (Kugler *et al.*, 1996). The higher ego-involvement of coaches might account for their pronounced response during soccer games: cortisol increases have been found to be more likely to be elicited by tasks demanding active performance of the participants (Dickerson and Kemeny, 2004), a condition certainly not met for supporters watching a game.

The goalless draw did not enable the testing of testosterone reactions against expected mood changes. The own team scoring a goal or the winning of the game were situations expected to be followed by positive mood changes (e.g. pride) whereas the opposite team scoring a goal or the game being lost were situations expected to be followed by negative mood changes (e.g. disappointment). Nevertheless, increases in testosterone coinciding with elevations in reported pride in a team's performance after the end of the game might be an interesting note in relation to Mazur and Lamb's (1980) suggestion of a link between testosterone and positive emotional states.

Future directions

Sport events can induce states of tension and even strong emotions, ranging from frustration to euphoric states. Some of these have been shown to lead to measurable changes in physiological parameters. The investigation of sport spectators should be seen as a promising field for researchers interested in looking at the psychophysiology of intense emotional states. Given the popularity of watching sports around the world, potential participants abound. Furthermore, no problems should arise concerning the ethical dilemma that researchers are often confronted with when wishing to induce negative emotions any other way.

In soccer games, goals usually signify the starting point of ecologically valid emotional states. The onset of both positive and negative emotional states can thus be sharply assigned to a certain point in time which is important for the assessment of elusive physiological reactions to them. For goals to provide a trigger for emotions that set themselves apart from the otherwise experienced emotional states, they need to happen infrequently. This is a criterion mostly met by soccer games, unlike basketball games, for example, which tend to have a much higher rate of scoring. Because for many parameters the changes in concentrations are usually measured with time lags of several minutes to the triggering event (e.g. Dickerson and Kemeny, 2004), it would be much more difficult to assign changes in the parameters to one specific scoring situation if goals or baskets are scored in rapid succession. In this case, the end of a game or a game-deciding situation might be a better choice than the scoring of any one basket. The best situation to select in order to capture situation-specific emotional states must be determined individually for each sport.

In general, in measuring the psychophysiology of emotional states in sports it would be best to choose situations with a sudden onset (i.e. clearly determinable with respect to time) and a significant impact on the outcome of a competition. The measuring of the parameters of interest should then take place immediately and in short intervals. It must be continued long enough to capture the reactions of the parameters usually reacting time-lagged to the triggering events.

The event-related data captured can then be compared with any other situation-specific data.

Most of the studies referred to in this chapter differentiate between victory and loss, and restrict measuring biological parameters to before and after the game. Whereas this measurement alignment might be adequate for spectators of a short competition such as, for example, an 800-m track and field run, it might not be for competitions lasting longer, such as soccer games. Here, emotions and potentially accompanying changes in hormonal concentrations evoked by game-deciding situations may not continue until collection points at the end of a competition. Because the samples needed to determine the parameters at focus request no specific preparation phase prior to collection, measurement points can very flexibly be introduced in an ongoing study. This way, assimilating a study's measurement alignment to the different courses a game or tournament might take becomes possible. Furthermore, the samples are not restrictively attached to certain places, but can easily be used in any sports stadium. Frequent measurement points will allow for more detailed physiological reaction profiles in the future. The measuring grid of the outlined pilot study revealed some interesting short-term changes that would have been missed if longer intervals had been set between measurement points.

The simultaneous consideration of two groups, each supporting one of two competing teams, would allow for investigation of the physiological profiles of diametrical opposed emotional states following goals or other game-deciding situations. The reported pilot study's priority was to find out more about the short-term on-line changes of different physiological parameters during a game. In a first step the attention was thus primarily aimed at the repeated measurement of the multiple parameters. Future studies should also consider including both control condition and supporters of the opposing team.

Reactions to sport events have been shown to depend on their characteristics, such as their outcomes or whether they are decided early on or hard fought until the end (Rose and Dunn, 1964; Bernhardt *et al.*, 1998; Carré and Putnam, 2010). Only the simultaneous consideration of different parameters therefore allows comparable conditions and enables differences in those parameters' sensitivity to an event or a psychological stressor to be detected. We can now investigate the interplay among biological systems, which will help clarify complex biological reaction patterns to stressors in more depth.

A last point deserves mention. The physiological reactions of competing athletes are understood as reactions to both the physiological stress of an athletic performance and the psychological stress accompanying a competitive situation. Some studies have been conducted to estimate the relative levels of athletes' physiological reactions to be ascribed to either psychological stress or physiological stress (e.g. Salvador *et al.*, 1987; Suay *et al.*, 1999). The investigation of sport spectators under laboratory conditions as described by Steiner *et al.* (2011) may be thought of another way to measure the physiological reactions attributable to competitive atmospheres found during sport events, and to provide some sort of reference upon which to compare active athletes' reaction profiles.

References

Bernhardt, P. C., Dabbs, J. M., Fielden, J. A. and Lutter, C. D. (1998). Testosterone changes during vicarious experiences of winning and losing among fans at sporting events. *Physiology and Behavior*, 65, 59–62.

Berthier, F. and Boulay, F. (2003). Lower myocardial infarction mortality in French men the day France won the 1998 World Cup of football. *Heart*, 89, 555–556.

Brunekreef, B. and Hoek, G. (2002). No association between major football games and cardiovascular mortality. *Epidemiology*, 13, 491–492.

Carré, J. M. and Putnam, S. K. (2010). Watching a previous victory produces an increase in testosterone among elite hockey players. *Psychoneuroendocrinology*, 35, 475–479.

Carroll, D., Ebrahim, S., Tilling, K., Macleod, J. and Smith, G. D. (2002). Admissions for myocardial infarction and World Cup football: database survey. *British Medical Journal*, 325, 1439–1442.

Dabbs, J. M. (1990). Salivary testosterone measurements: reliability across hours, days, and weeks. *Physiology and Behavior*, 48, 83–86.

Dickerson, S. S. and Kemeny, M. E. (2004). Acute stressors and cortisol responses: a theoretical integration and synthesis of laboratory research. *Psychological Bulletin*, 130, 355–391.

Edwards, D. A., Wetzel, K. and Wyner, D. R. (2006). Intercollegiate soccer: saliva cortisol and testosterone are elevated during competition, and testosterone is related to status and social connectedness with teammates. *Physiology and Behavior*, 87, 135–143.

Harrison, L. K., Carroll, D., Burns, V. E., *et al.* (2000). Cardiovascular and secretory immunoglobulin A reactions to humorous, exciting, and didactic film presentations. *Biological Psychology*, 52, 113–126.

Hirt, E. R., Zillmann, D., Erickson, G. A. and Kennedy, C. (1992). Costs and benefits of allegiance: changes in fans' self-ascribed competencies after team victory versus defeat. *Journal of Personality and Social Psychology*, 63, 724–738.

Hijzen, T. H. and Slangen, J. L. (1985). The electrocardiogram during emotional and physical stress. *International Journal of Psychophysiology*, 2, 273–279.

Hüllemann, K. D., Mayer, H. and Stahlheber, R. (1971). Fernsehen und herz-kreislaufregulation kreislaufuntersuchungen bei herzinfarktpatienten und normalpersonen während der fernsehübertragung von fussballweltmeisterschaftsspielen. [Television and cardiovascular regulation. Circulation studies on myocardial infarct patients and subjects with normal findings during the television transmission of soccer world championship games]. *Münchener Medizinische Wochenschrift*, 113, 1401–1406.

Katz, E., Metzger, J. T., Marazzi, A. and Kappenberger, L. (2006). Increase of sudden cardiac deaths in Switzerland during the 2002 FIFA World Cup. *International Journal of Cardiology*, 107, 132–133.

Katz, E., Metzger, J. T., Schlaepfer, J., *et al.* (2005). Increase of out-of-hospital cardiac arrests in the male population of the French speaking provinces of Switzerland during the 1998 FIFA World Cup. *Heart*, 91, 1096–1097.

Kugler, J., Reintjes, F., Tewes, V. and Schedlowski, M. (1996). Competition stress in soccer coaches increases salivary immunoglobulin A and salivary cortisol concentrations. *Journal of Sports Medicine and Physical Fitness*, 36, 117–120.

Mazur, A. and Lamb, T. A. (1980). Testosterone, status, and mood in human males. *Hormones and Behavior*, 14, 236–246.

Rose, K. D. and Dunn, F. L. (1964). The heart of the spectator sportsman. *Medical Times*, 92, 945–951.

Salvador, A., Simòn, V., Suay, F. and Llorens, L. (1987). Testosterone and cortisol responses to competitive fighting in human males: a pilot study. *Aggressive Behavior*, 13, 9–13.

Schwarz, N., Strack, F., Kammer, D. and Wagner, D. (1987). Soccer, rooms, and the quality of your life: mood effects on judgements of satisfaction with life in general and with specific domains. *European Journal of Social Psychology*, 17, 69–79.

Sloan, L.R. (1979). The function and impact of sports for fans: review of theory and contemporary research. In J. H. Goldstein (ed.), *Sports, Games, and Play* (pp. 219–269). Hillsdale, NJ: Erlbaum.

Steiner, S., Abbruzzese, E., La Marca, R. and Ehlert, U. (2011). Autonomic stress responses elicited by watching a live broadcast soccer game: a pilot study. Manuscript submitted for publication.

Suay, F., Salvador, A., González-Bono, E., *et al.* (1999). Effects of competition and its outcome on serum testosterone, cortisol, and prolactin. *Psychoneuroendocrinology*, 24, 551–566.

Tegelman, R., Carlström, K. and Pousette, Å. (1988). Hormone levels in male ice hockey players during a 26-hour cup tournament. *International Journal of Andrology*, 11, 361–368.

Task Force of the European Society and Cardiology and the North American Society of Pacing and Electrophysiology (1996). Heart rate variability. Standards of measurements, physiological interpretation, and clinical use. *European Heart Journal*, 17, 354–381.

Van Stegeren, A., Rohleder, N., Everaerd, W. and Wolf, O. T. (2006). Salivary alpha amylase as marker for adrenergic activity during stress: effect of betablockade. *Psychoneuroendocrinology*, 31, 137–141.

Witte, D. R., Bots, M. L., Hoes, A. W. and Grobbee, D. E. (2000). Cardiovascular mortality in Dutch men during 1996 European football championship: longitudinal study. *British Medical Journal*, 321, 1552–1554.

10 Staleness and the overtraining syndrome

Ferran Suay

Although competition is the best-known sports activity, sports practitioners devote the most part of their time to quite a different kind of activity: training. Sports training is a progressive adaptive process of a non-linear nature, aimed to maximally increase the probability of achieving great performances, by means of sequentially assigning workloads and recovery periods (Rowbottom and Green, 2000; Bonete and Suay, 2003). Thus, the training process involves successive and planned acute efforts aimed to disturb homeostasis and create fatigue in order to evoke an adaptive response of the organism at various levels, which would lead to an increased ability to sustain either a maximal or submaximal intensity for a longer time than the rivals. Every one of these efforts (training loads) may be considered as an acute stressor, while the whole training schedule – with its dynamic balance between effort and recovery – constitutes a good example of a chronic stressor to which sports performers would have to adapt. The ability to cope with both kinds of stressors is central to the process of achieving higher performance levels.

Training schedules of high-level performers in many specialities are time-consuming, tiring and hard to undertake. In general, high levels of motivation are needed to complete the daily training programmes throughout the whole training and competition season. One of the essential abilities needed to achieve and maintain a high level of sports performance is an enhanced capacity to tolerate fatigue and even to ignore its most salient symptoms, including pain and lack of motivation. Without this capacity it is doubtful that anyone would be able to be in the sports-world elite, at least in the most physically demanding specialities. It is worth noting that those very demanding training schedules are not, nowadays, exclusive to elite performers. Many ambitious young athletes may be willing to intensify their training loads in an attempt to improve their competitive status and join the elite. Frequently they are not subjected to strict coach supervision or medical control (in some cases, they may even be self-training) and may run a high risk of suffering the negative consequences of overtraining.

In recent decades training schedules have increased dramatically in most competitive sports. Bompa (1983) stated that from 1975 to 1980 increases in yearly training hours for many sports ranged from 10% to 22% and this tendency seems to have been intensified since then (Kenttä et al., 2001; Meeusen, et al., 2006; Matos et al., 2011). As an example, the former 1972 Olympic seven gold-medal winner Mark Spitz covered daily distances of about 9 km. Although this is a very impressive training load, many Olympic swimmers are nowadays performing 36 km per day (Peterson, 2005). Together with the introduction of full-body swim suits (now banned in swimming contests), those highly intensified training schedules may have contributed to the dramatic progresses achieved during the last years. Records have been broken time and again in quite spectacular and celebrated ways. Moreover, elite performers have become internationally well known and many of them have earned significant amounts of money.

However, such impressive training loads do not always lead to enhanced benefits. When inadequate training stress is applied and/or recovery time is insufficient, performance reduction and chronic maladaptation occurs. Known as overtraining syndrome (OTS), this complex condition afflicts people engaged in demanding training schedules. The prevalence of OTS in specific sports is difficult to establish. In the few studies available, incidence rates for athletes have ranged between 10 and 64% in individual sports, and between 33 and 50% in team sports (Kenttä et al., 2001). For elite runners, for example, two studies (Morgan et al., 1987, 1988) stated that 60% of women and 64% of men reported having experienced a bout of staleness at least once during their running career. In contrast, only 33% of non-elite women runners had experienced staleness.

Although OTS in young athletes may be a major obstacle on their road to success, there is little information about OTS prevalence in young and aspiring elite athletes (Kenttä et al., 2001). Incidence rates of 35% have been reported in young swimmers from several countries, with ages ranging between 13 and 18 years (Raglin et al. 2000). In team sports, 33% of the athletes in a basketball team developed staleness during a six-week training period, while more than 50% of the football players in a team were similarly affected during the first four months of their competitive season (Kenttä et al., 2001).

The main criticisms on the reliability of those data are related to the use of unclear classifications to distinguish between overtrained and non-overtrained subjects. Moreover, it has to be considered that many cases of OTS are not reported in any way if they are suffered by athletes of lower competitive levels, or even if the sports performers and/or their technical staffs are not willing to inform about them. Nevertheless, the performance- and health-harming consequences of such a condition are dramatic enough to merit a high level of interest among sports scientists and professionals, and suggest that we should increase our knowledge of overtraining processes and of the ways to prevent underperformance.

Despite a number of scientific investigations, the underlying mechanisms of overtraining are still poorly understood and no objective biomarkers for overtraining have been identified. Partially as a consequence of this, a great deal of research has been conducted focusing on psychological markers of the overtraining process which may provide a good degree of usefulness. There is also a promising line of investigation centred on immunological markers (see Purvis et al., 2010 for a review). However, the present chapter will focus on hormonal markers in order to provide useful information for sports psychologists about what they can do to monitor training and prevent underperformance.

Overtraining, overreaching and overtraining syndrome

Since there is some inconsistency in the terminology used in the scientific literature, we will try to clarify the terms that will appear here. The term *overtraining* has
been defined as 'an accumulation of training and non-training stress resulting in a
long-term decrement in performance capacity with or without related physiological and psychological signs and symptoms of overtraining in which restoration of
performance may take from several weeks to months' (Kreider *et al.*, 1998). This
is a general definition which includes the process ('accumulation of training and
non-training stress') as well as the outcome ('long-term decrement in performance capacity'). It is important to establish a clear distinction between the process
and the outcome because every athlete is subjected to overtraining dynamics. If
they are willing to improve their competitive performances, the athletes have to
train and then they have to train further (to overtrain). In this sense, the term
should not be given a pathological connotation.

On the other hand, when the consequence of such a process of intensified
training is maladaptation and health deterioration, we are speaking about a non-
desired pathological state that should receive some other name. The *overtraining
syndrome* is a sports phenomenon that can be produced by physical, emotional,
psychological and social stressors and that evokes responses that can be observed
and eventually assessed on all these levels.

The name of the syndrome implies that excess exercise is the sole causative factor, whereas, although an imbalance between training and recovery seems to be
the primary cause of this dysfunction, many other factors related to the athlete's
personal, familiar, social or professional environments may play a role and its
aetiology appears multifactorial. Because of its seemingly causal implications, it
has been proposed that OTS should be called *unexplained underperformance syndrome* (UPS). This has been defined as a persistent decrease in athletic performance capacity, despite two weeks of relative rest (Budgett *et al.*, 2000). Since this
generic denomination does not assume causation or responsibility for trainers, the
term UPS might be preferred. Nevertheless, the scientific literature has mostly
concentrated on the relationships between training loads and physiological, psychological and performance consequences, while other stress sources have not
been so widely investigated. For that reason we will keep using the term overtraining syndrome (OTS) for the maladaptive state resulting from the accumulation of
training and non-training stress.

It is also necessary to differentiate OTS from *overreaching* (also called *short-term
overtraining*), which has been defined as 'an accumulation of training and/or non-
training stress resulting in short-term decrement in performance capacity with or
without related physiological and psychological signs and symptoms of maladaptation in which restoration of performance capacity may take from several days to
several weeks' (Kreider *et al.*, 1998). The state in which athletes experience 'short
term performance decrement, without severe psychological, or lasting other negative symptoms' may be labelled as *functional overreaching* (FOR) and will eventually
lead to an improvement in performance after recovery (Meeusen *et al.*, 2006).

On the other hand, if the balance between training and recovery is not suf-ficiently respected, *non-functional overreaching* (NFOR) can occur. It is worth noting 'the distinction between NFOR and the Overtraining Syndrome (OTS) is very difficult and will depend on the clinical outcome and exclusion diagno-sis. The athlete will often show the same clinical, hormonal and other signs and symptoms' (Meeusen *et al.*, 2006, p. 3).

As the aforementioned definitions suggest, the important differential between overtraining and overreaching may be the amount of time needed for performance restoration, more than the degree of impairment (Budgett *et al.*, 2000; Halson and Jeukendrup, 2004). On the other hand, OTS is considered to be an exceptional (not desired) condition and the term 'overtrained' should be used for people in heavy training losing performance without an obvious clinical reason which is sustained for more than two weeks (Lehmann *et al.*, 1999).

The borderline between optimal performance and performance impairment due to OTS is subtle. This applies especially to physiological and biochemical factors (Meeusen *et al.*, 2006) and diagnosis of OTS is further complicated by the fact that the clinical features show a high inter-individual variation.

It has been repeatedly suggested that OTS could be broken into sympathetic and parasympathetic classifications (Lehmann *et al.*, 1993, 1999; Kellmann, 2002). The sympathetic form would be associated with more easily identifiable symptoms such as increased heart rate and blood pressure, decreased appetite, loss of body weight, irritability and disturbed sleep. It is less frequent and sup-posedly affects mostly anaerobic sports such as sprinting, jumping and throwing. In contrast, the parasympathetic form would go with lowered resting heart rate and blood pressure, excessive sleep and behavioural inhibition or even depression (Kellmann, 2002). This purportedly affects highly trained endurance athletes in mostly aerobic sports such as long-distance running, swimming and road cycling (Armstrong and Van Heest, 2002).

The distinction appears conceptually clear and attractive since the physical demands of intense, short-term efforts are widely different from the ones pro-voked by long-lasting, endurance efforts. Nevertheless, the research findings do not support this distinction and it is not even certain that the anaerobic versus aerobic distinction holds up well. Moreover, it has to be taken into account that endurance athletes also undertake significant amounts of resistance training in the same way that sprinters and other mostly anaerobic performers carry out sig-nificant amounts of endurance training. Thus, although the energetic demands of endurance (i.e. a marathon race) and resistance sports (i.e. a 100-metre race) may be very different in competition, the training schedules of both types of athletes may share a great deal of common activities. It would be difficult to answer the question about which of the two types of training should be held responsible for an eventual OTS.

To summarize, according to the ECSS Task Force consensus statement (Meeusen *et al.*, 2006), the term 'overtraining' should be understood as a proc-ess of intensified training with three possible outcomes: short-term overreach-ing (functional), extreme overreaching (non-functional) or OTS. The usage of

PROCESS	TRAINING (overload)	INTENSIFIED TRAINING →		
OUTCOME	ACUTE FATIGUE	FUNCTIONAL OR (short-term OR)	NON-FUNCTIONAL OVERREACHING (extreme OR)	OVERTRAINING SYNDROM (OTS)
RECOVERY	Day(s)	Days – weeks	Weeks – months	Months – ...
PERFORMANCE	INCREASE	Temporary performance decrement (e.g. training camp)	STAGNATION DECREASE	DECREASE

Figure 10.1 Description of the relation between intensity of training and the different stages of training, overreaching and the overtraining syndrome. Reprinted from Meeusen *et al.* (2006). Prevention, diagnosis and treatment of the Over-training Syndrome. *European Journal of Sport Science*, 6(1), 1–14, with permission of Taylor & Francis Ltd.

'syndrome' is purposeful. It acknowledges that exercise (training) is not neces-sarily the sole causative factor of the maladaptive state and also emphasizes its multifactorial aetiology during competition or training. Figure 10.1 presents the stages that differentiate normal training from overreaching (functional and non-functional overreaching) and from the OTS.

In summary, we can consider that most sports performers are subjected to overtraining (meaning that they have to intensify their training schedules). Some of them may reach a borderline state – overreaching – that is neither entirely pathologic nor completely maladaptive (it may be reached intention-ally in order to get a maximum increase in performance), but that takes the athletes to the limits of their adaptive capacity. Otherwise, when athletes fail to achieve great performances as a consequence of their demanding training schedules (and probably also because of the influence of other stressors) and experience a variety of signs and symptoms that accompany the performance deterioration, it may be said that those athletes are overtrained or suffering an OTS.

Hormonal markers

Although our knowledge of the central pathological mechanisms of the OTS has significantly improved in recent years, there is still a strong demand for reliable tools (markers) for the early diagnosis of OTS. The interest of sports scientists and practitioners in this field has focused on identifying valid early warning signals that allow them to know whether – at any specific moment – the athletes are able to tolerate the training loads they are undertaking or whether their adaptive capacity is being seriously compromised. The sooner in the process they have this knowledge, the better they will be able to modulate the training loads in order to prevent undesired underperformance.

Since 'early and unequivocal recognition of OTS is virtually impossible because the only certain sign is a decrease in performance' (Meeusen *et al.*, 2006), the most commonly accepted markers of OTS are drops in performance or the inability to train at customary levels. There are, nevertheless, three main problems associated with those signs: (1) they may appear, albeit temporarily, in well-adapting individuals, (2) they may not be obvious until the athlete is severely affected by OTS and (3) it is not clear how much performance has to drop to indicate an OTS. The signs therefore lack the two main characteristics of a valid marker: sensitivity and specificity. Clearly, it is not advisable to rely entirely on these markers, and coaches and sport professionals still need some useful criteria to reliably titrate training schedules according to the actual evolution of their athletes' adaption. The definition of OTS should be restricted to actual decreases in performance. Thus, the hormonal measures should be used in addition to a battery of screening tools (Halson and Jeukendrup, 2004).

Although over 250 symptoms of OTS have been listed, the most commonly reported symptoms include elevated resting heart rate, weight loss, sleep and mood disturbances (including depression of clinical significance), and chronic fatigue (Fry *et al.*, 1991). Again, the main problem is to ascertain whether the occurrence of any of these symptoms is unambiguously indicating the onset of an OTS or only signalling overreaching, which, as previously stated, may be a desired outcome. Thus, an inability to clearly separate overtrained from non-overtrained athletes is a main weakness of the overtraining scientific literature and in many studies, athletes have been classified as overtrained (or stale) based on vague definitions of OTS.

These are important reasons that have instigated the search for more objective markers of overtraining. Many different types of indices have been studied in an attempt to provide useful tools to prevent underperformance. Since it has been hypothesized that a hormonal-mediated central malfunction occurs during the pathogenesis of the OTS (Fry *et al.*, 1991; Meeusen *et al.*, 2006), the measurement of blood hormones has been favoured by many research teams.

Why hormonal markers?

The inherent logic of relying on hormonal markers to monitor training adaptation appears conceptually solid. If an organism has to adapt to increasingly demanding workloads, the endocrine system will have to experience some changes which allow it to undertake the challenge. Its stress response will have to progress in order to be able to overcome the progressively greater stressors included in the training schedule. That should affect the two main stress response systems, so provoking changes in the production of the stress-related hormones.

As stated earlier, training is a process in which work and recovery should be combined in order to enhance physical performance. Thus, the catabolic processes triggered and sustained by hormones such as catecholamines and cortisol in order to provide the required energy should be compensated by anabolic processes. The anabolism is carried out during the recovery periods and benefits from the cellular actions of sexual steroids. An improved physical condition would only be achieved if effort-depleted energetic stores are replenished and broken fibre muscles are replaced by other, stronger, well-adapted ones. Since the endocrine system is considered as a second-intention regulatory system with roles in the production and maintenance of adaptations, the measurement of hormones may provide useful information about an athlete's adaptive status. These measures may be most useful when taken together with information on performance, training load and psychological responses (Urhausen and Kindermann, 2002).

Which hormonal markers?

It has to be stated that hormones are only a possible surrogate marker of overreaching/overtraining. The available knowledge does not permit us to assert that any given amount or change of a specific hormone unequivocally signals the presence of a pathological state such as OTS. Thus, a current diagnosis of overreaching or overtraining would most probably rely on the measurement of performance reduction and clinical symptoms. Nevertheless, since hormonal concentrations may provide useful information, cortisol, testosterone-to-cortisol ratio (T/C) and catecholamine concentrations will be discussed below.

Resting cortisol

At the hormonal level, physical exercise is a type of allostatic load for various endocrine systems (McEwen and Lasley, 2003), notably the HPA axis. The primary product of this axis, the catabolic hormone cortisol, plays an important role in energetic metabolism by stimulating the catabolic processes needed to obtain energy from the available substrates. Its response is affected by all kinds of stressful situations, including training loads and sports competitions (Suay and Salvador, 2003) and it is considered that resting cortisol concentrations generally reflect a long-term training stress (Kraemer and Ratamess, 2005) and could provide useful information about possible dysfunction of the HPA axis (Steinacker *et al.*, 2004; Gouarné *et al.*, 2005).

Among other consequences, during heavy training periods, the predominance of catabolic processes would explain the fact that both an increase in muscular discomfort and a pronounced weight loss are described in the literature as signs associated with states of severe fatigue, which may often go together with performance decrements (Hawley and Schoene, 2003; Steinacker *et al.*, 2004; Lac and Maso, 2004).

Although cortisol responses have been widely studied in relation to training adaptation, the results are far from conclusive. Some studies have reported decreases, while others have found cortisol increases in overtrained subjects, or even in well-adapted athletes. Others have failed to find significant changes after intensity or volume increases, or have reported variable cortisol responses (Hedelin *et al.*, 2000). Although it has been proposed that volume and/or training intensity increases would provoke cortisol increases as a consequence of the higher physiological strain endured (Urhausen *et al.*, 1998), resting cortisol cannot be considered as an unequivocal marker of training adaptation or of failure to adapt (Urhausen and Kindermann, 2002).

Testosterone-to-cortisol ratio (T/C)

Like cortisol, testosterone production is dependent on the hypothalamic–pituitary system and testosterone constitutes the final product of the hypothalamic–pituitary–gonadal (HPG) axis. In contrast to cortisol, testosterone is the main anabolic hormone. In men it is endogenously produced by testicular Leydig cells while in women, who produce significantly lower amounts of this steroid, it is secreted by the adrenal cortex upon ACTH stimulation. Testosterone cellular actions are in opposition to those of cortisol and are oriented to increase protein synthesis, thus contributing to muscle mass gains among other restorative processes.

The HPA and HPG axes are closely linked. HPG axis influences on the HPA axis are both organizing effects during fetal life and activating effects of sex hormones in adult life. Such mechanisms are thought to account for the higher prevalence of mood disorders in women as compared to men. In addition, the stress system is affected by changing levels of sex hormones, as found, for example, during the premenstrual period, ante- and postpartum, during the transition phase to the menopause and during the use of oral contraceptives. In depressed women, plasma levels of oestrogen are usually lower and plasma levels of androgens are increased, while testosterone levels are decreased in depressed men (Schwab *et al.*, 2005). It may be interesting to remember, at this point, that one of the most prevalent symptoms observed in overtrained athletes is mood deterioration, including clinical depression (Suay *et al.*, 1998).

In the other direction, it can be said that activation of the HPA axis leads to a decrease in HPG activity and so to a reduced testosterone secretion. All kinds of stressors act on the HPG axis by decreasing circulating levels of gonadotrophins. This outcome is associated with increased activation of the HPA axis. So, the well-known role of the resulting elevation in circulating glucocorticoids to overcome the challenge to homeostasis also acts on the HPG axis to reduce sex hormone secretion. Although the inherent mechanism is not well understood, exogenous glucocorticoids have been shown to suppress gonadotrophin secretion, which is one of the first steps in the hormonal cascade leading to testosterone production (Schwab *et al.*, 2005).

Considering the systemic relationship between the two final products of the HPA and HPG axes, there seems to be a good reason to look at their dynamic balance in the bloodstream in order to assess the degree of adaptation to a chronic stressor such as training. The relative concentrations of testosterone and cortisol should indicate a balance between anabolic and catabolic effects and it is easy to conclude that for progress to occur a slight (at least) predominance of anabolism has to be present. Otherwise, if destructive processes are prevalent in an organism's internal milieu it would seem odd to predict any performance increases.

On these grounds, an early study suggested that overtraining could be related to a significant decrease in testosterone, or at least of the ratio between testosterone and cortisol (Adlercreutz *et al.*, 1986). Since then, the testosterone/cortisol (T/C) ratio and/or free testosterone/cortisol ratio (fT/C) have been proposed as feasible indicators of the anabolic/catabolic status of skeletal muscle during training. It is considered that a decrease in testosterone, an increase in cortisol or both would indicate a potential state of excessive catabolism that should not be compatible with the correct adaptations that may lead to enhanced performance.

Two different criteria were proposed for the T/C. The absolute one states that a value lower than 0.35×10^{-3} (testosterone measured in nmol/L and cortisol in mmol/L) would indicate an overtrained state (Adlercreutz *et al.*, 1986), whereas the second one suggests that decreases larger than 30% of the previous basal values are a condition for the diagnosis of an overtrained state (Urhausen *et al.*, 1995). Application of both criteria has resulted in a great deal of practical and methodological difficulties and inconsistencies related to the different methods used to analyse and determine hormone concentrations and also to the feasibility of using this index in different athletic specialities and in both sexes (Suay *et al.*, 1997).

Moreover, despite a considerable volume of research, the results are disappointing. Some studies have shown changes in the T/C ratio during strength and power training, and this ratio has been positively related to performance improvements, whereas other studies have shown no change. Most of the studies have been unable to confirm changes in the T/C ratio in overtrained endurance or strength athletes (Urhausen and Kindermann, 2002). In an animal study where the T/C ratio was manipulated to investigate muscle hypertrophy, it was reported that this index was not a useful indicator of tissue anabolism. Thus, the utility of the T/C ratio remains controversial (Kraemer and Ratamess, 2005) and it has been suggested that the ratio would actually indicate the physiological strain of training rather than a maladaptive (overtrained) state (Urhausen and Kindermann, 2002).

Catecholamines

Since the importance of the sympathetic nervous system for adaptation of stress and the relationship between physical training and the activity of the sympathetic nervous system are well accepted, catecholamine secretion has been studied in relation to overtraining.

Catecholamines reflect the acute demands of the training load and are important for increasing force production, muscle contraction rate, energy availability, as well as several other functions, including the increases of hormones such as testosterone. All of these actions are involved in performance enhancement.

Two different parameters may be considered in catecholamine concentrations: (a) the acute response to a specific effort and (b) the resting levels.

Catecholamine secretion is very sensitive to homeostatic disruption. The mere act of standing causes a dramatic increase in plasma concentrations of these hormones and acute bouts of exercise increase plasma concentrations of catecholamines in a magnitude dependent upon different exercise characteristics (e.g. force of muscle contraction, amount of muscle stimulated, volume of exercise and rest intervals). Adrenaline is secreted in greater amounts than noradrenaline and dopamine and even prior to intense exercise, an anticipatory rise consisting in significant elevations in plasma adrenaline and noradrenaline is produced. This anticipatory rise is considered to be part of the body's psychophysiological adjustment for preparing to maximally perform. Although chronic adaptations remain unclear, it has been suggested that training reduces the catecholamine response to resistance exercise, so revealing an adaptive process since the same work can be performed with a lower catecholamine concentration (Kraemer and Ratamess, 2005). Conversely, poorly adapted individuals would need more of these hormones to carry out the same effort.

Thus, catecholamines concentrations in response to a standard effort may be used to assess adaptation. Again, difficulties arise when considering quantitative criteria. As with other hormones, the extraordinarily high inter-individual variability prevents an unequivocal distinction between well-adapting and over-reached subjects.

For basal values, the logic is quite different. Excretion of catecholamines in the urine is considered to be an integrative indicator of total production and excretion of catecholamines over 24 hours. The rate at which the adrenal gland produces catecholamines may be considered an indicator of the sympathoadrenal system's capacity for stress response. So, it is thought that an impaired catecholamine production – manifested by low catecholamine concentrations – should indicate a decreased capacity to cope with stress and, thus, a maladaptive state resulting from adrenal exhaustion (Mackinnon *et al.*, 1997). In agreement with this statement, basal urinary catecholamine excretion has been reported to be significantly reduced in overtrained athletes (Lehmann *et al.*, 1992a). Moreover, a decreased nocturnal urinary excretion of catecholamines – interpreted as lowered intrinsic sympathetic activity – has been suggested as a rather late sign of OTS in overtrained athletes (Lehmann *et al.*, 1992b; Mackinnon *et al.*, 1997). The results obtained, however, are not conclusive and some investigations have not confirmed decreased nocturnal urine excretion of catecholamine (Urhausen and Kindermann, 2002). This lack of consistency may be related to methodological differences and high inter-individual differences in catecholamine responses to exercise. The collection method (urinary 24-hour or nocturnal excretion) employed to measure the autonomic nervous system activity and also the different analytic techniques may contribute to making comparison between the measures obtained more difficult.

While 24-hour catecholamine excretion or nocturnal urinary excretion are often considered more valid measures, catecholamine responses to an exercise challenge can give additional information on autonomic nervous system responses to exercise. Very often the selection of one of these methods depends on practical issues, including which one best fits the training schedules and the willingness of coaches and athletes to engage with the sampling protocols.

How are the samples collected?

In order to implement a method for gathering hormonal information from an individual athlete or a training group it is advisable to avoid invasive measures such as blood sampling. Fortunately, there are valid alternatives to hormone concentrations determination in blood nowadays. Saliva and urine sampling provide good available alternatives which have been repeatedly tested in training and competition contexts (Salvador, 2005).

Cortisol and testosterone in saliva

Saliva sampling is a reliable method for determining cortisol and testosterone concentrations. Salivary levels accurately reflect the unbound, biologically active, fractions of these hormones in general circulation (Granger and Kivlighan, 2003). Blood sampling – an invasive and somewhat annoying method – has an important drawback for the determination of hormonal concentrations in training sets: only a limited number of samples can be obtained from a subject with this procedure and some subjects may be reluctant to provide blood samples. So, saliva sampling represents a simple, non-invasive and stress-free measure that can greatly facilitate studies carried out on sport practitioners.

Saliva may be obtained via two different collection methods:

- by passive drooling in which subjects are asked to wash their mouth with distilled water; followed by a 2-minute dribble and spit, and a further 4-minute dribble collection in plastic tubes; or
- by the collection of saliva carried out using Salivette tampons. Participants are required to place a cotton dental roll in their mouth for approximately 30 seconds and then to put it in a plastic tube.

In both cases, samples may be collected at home, at training sets, or elsewhere and stored at room temperature or in the refrigerator until delivery to the laboratory. In both cases, saliva samples can be stored at $-20°C$ until they are processed to determine hormone concentrations. This kind of mailing procedure has been shown not to affect the hormones concentration and the samples can be stored frozen for up to at least two years without compromising sample integrity.

In order to assess the athlete's adaptation to training programmes, saliva samples should be collected at the same time of the day and in non-effort conditions. Since cortisol is affected not only by physical effort but also by psychological stressors and fasting, the sampling conditions would benefit from being as standardized as possible. Awakening time is suitable since it follows the longer daily resting period. Moreover, the cortisol-awakening response (CAR), a term which describes the rapid increase in cortisol levels following morning awakening, is considered a well-substantiated measure of the HPA axis basal activity (Kudielka and Wüst, 2010). If choosing this measure it should be taken into account that each participant will have to collect two saliva samples in every sampling day – the first one immediately on awakening then another one after a period usually ranging from 15 to 45 minutes post-awakening.

Other possibilities are available and it is always necessary to take into account the multiple conditions affecting cortisol and testosterone circulating levels. Circadian rhythms, physical exertion and exposure to psychological stressors are among the most important factors affecting both hormones and have to be considered in selecting appropriate sampling times.

Catecholamine concentrations in urine

Catecholamine concentrations can be determined in urine. Since in training contexts, catecholamine determinations are usually aimed at studying the adaptation of the athletes to the whole training programme and not their response to a specific training load, a global measure of catecholamine excretion may be preferred. There are two main ways to collect urine in order to assess catecholamine excretion: 24-hour urine samples and nocturnal urinary catecholamine excretion (NUCE).

- *24-hour urine samples*: the athletes should be provided with collection containers to collect their urine. To preserve the substance to be tested, the container may need to be refrigerated during the entire collection process. After getting up in the morning, the subjects should empty their bladders, discard that urine and note the time. For the next 24 hours, they will be asked to save all urine voided in the container provided. When 24 hours are over, they should empty their bladders and add this urine to the container, also noting the time. All of the urine collected has to be brought to the laboratory as soon as possible. The problem with this procedure is that catecholamine concentrations will be affected strongly by the training loads. Thus, it is advisable to gather these urine samples in a resting day, with athletes having refrained from training for at least 12 hours. This condition is not always suitable or well accepted by athletes and coaches.
- *Nocturnal urinary catecholamine excretion (NUCE)*: an overnight urine sample has to be obtained from each athlete. Usually, urine would be collected after 10 p.m. the previous night (the 10 p.m. void discarded) up to and including the first void in the morning. Urine is collected in specially designed plastic bottles containing a chemical solvent, and stored at 4°C by the subject until transferred to the laboratory. Often HCl is used as the preservative in urine samples to prevent microbial contamination.

In the measurement of urinary parameters, various preservatives (HCl, $NaHCO_3$, boric acid, chlorhexidine, etc.) are used for different purposes such as prevention of bacterial growth, stability of metabolites etc. (Yilmaz *et al.*, 2008).

Unlike blood sampling, both saliva and NUCE sampling methods are non-invasive procedures that can be implemented in groups of athletes without significantly harming their training schedules. Since NUCE sampling does not interfere with training routines it will probably be the first choice for athletes and coaches.

How many samples?

According to the state of the art in the field of hormonal markers of overtraining no single hormonal value is considered able to provide a valid diagnostic. It does not mean that hormonal markers are useless. In some circumstances and with all the due cautions they may provide useful information, giving a complementary perspective on athletes' adaptive status.

The best method would be a large sampling which allows one to set basal lines. Ideally it should be maintained throughout the whole sports season. Comparison of the hormone values observed during a critical training period with those obtained during rest periods or during regular (non-intensive) training days, together with the consideration of other indicators (mood states, training performances, signs and symptoms, an athlete's personal communications, etc.) may contribute to an understanding of their actual adaptive or maladaptive status. A significant problem for practitioners is determining which baseline values are the most appropriate. Is it during the rest period (no training) or should it be when the athletes are clearly coping well with their training loads?

Advantages and disadvantages of hormonal markers

Measuring hormones may provide information about an athlete's inner adaptation to training programmes. Unlike psychological data obtained through tests and interviews, hormonal data are not easily biased, even if an individual's intention is to eventually hide his or her maladaptive condition. This is a most inadvisable and undesired intention but professionals working in high level sports know that some performers would be reluctant to reveal their actual condition for various reasons, including their strong motivation to take part in selected competitive events and their fear of being discarded. If accurately collected, analysed and interpreted, the measurement of hormone levels would provide a complementary approach, helping coaches and athletes to make the right decisions about intensifying subsequent training loads or not.

Admittedly, the collection of hormone information is not completely without effort or costs. These are relatively expensive methods of monitoring and although saliva or urine collection procedures are clearly better and easier than blood sampling, they are not without difficulty and inconvenience.

The day-to-day variation in hormones may be another concern since mental stress, physical activity, diet and sleep patterns are known to significantly alter hormone concentrations in blood. These factors could affect them during the period of blood collections and thus have to be considered. Repeated measures analysis of variances may be used to test for differences within each hormone across days, and intraclass correlations (ICC) and typical error is useful to assess the reliability of hormone concentrations across days. Results have revealed resting hormonal values within accepted clinical ranges. A study conducted in exercise-trained men (Hackney and Zack, 2006) suggests that resting testosterone and cortisol concentrations are not highly variable and appear to be reliable from day to day in exercise-trained men.

Other factors to consider are that the athletes will have to assume responsibility for collection on schedule and for temporary storage of the samples. They will have to master a clearly explained sampling protocol and – as has been said – a certain amount of money will have to be allocated in order to get the information. Nevertheless, there are circumstances under which it may be worth doing and there are training groups that may be able to afford the costs and to overcome the practical challenges. World-class elite athletes in extremely demanding disciplines may be willing to undertake the burdens of applying this methodology in order to get a better insight into their development and some helpful information which allows coaches and doctors to make the right decisions about training loads.

The main disadvantage is the lack of clear-cut diagnostic criteria to distinguish between well-adapted and overtrained (maladapted) athletes. The fast turnaround in laboratory testing of these measures also contributes to this difficulty in establishing consistent and reliable quantitative criteria for hormonal markers. Moreover, the distinction between overreached (a temporary maladaptive state) and overtrained (a chronic maladaptive state) is crucial and again there are no valid criteria for this.

An additional difficulty is that a wide sampling in normal (non-overtraining) conditions will be needed from every athlete. Since no available evidence supports the use of hormones for delineating between overreached and overtrained athletes, a multifactorial approach is suggested for OTS diagnosis (Brink *et al.*, 2010). Nevertheless, significant differences between hormonal levels obtained in critical training periods and those 'normal values' may act as a clue that a maladaptive state is developing.

Final considerations and future directions

Training control procedures are most effective if they are designed and implemented by the whole technical staff. Coaches and doctors, along with psychologists, can create or adapt better training control strategies while working together and sharing information. For sport psychologists it is usual to include information obtained from psychological testing but (perhaps after reading this book) they may also be willing to gather hormonal information.

In order to include hormonal variables among their strategies of training control technical staff need to consider some important points. In some cases these will be the same as in other procedures, such as psychological testing (testing conditions, confidentiality), but there are also some specific factors that are briefly addressed here.

Approaching coaches

Although it is difficult to find an adjective deriving from the term 'unexplained underperformance syndrome', we consider it advisable to use it when speaking with coaches or athletes. Not implying any causal reason for the observed (or avoided) maladaptive state and their professional practice may lead coaches to feel more comfortable and more willing to cooperate. It should be made clear that the proposed procedures are intended to prevent undesired or unexplained underperformance.

Previous information

Athletes and coaches should be clearly informed about the characteristics of the hormonal measures to be taken. It may be useful to state that these are not doping-control measures and that the results are strictly for the use of the technical staff and will not be available for any other person. Moreover, it is recommended that a written informed consent should be signed by every participant.

Circadian rhythms

Since hormones are subjected to biological variations along a 24-hour cycle (circadian comes from the Latin *circa diem*, meaning 'more or less one day'), samples should always be collected at the same time of the day in order to allow valid comparisons.

Results interpretation

Since most sport psychologists do not have the necessary biology background to fully understand the significance of hormonal values, it is advisable to collaborate with medical doctors. Of course, it is also a valid alternative to get the necessary knowledge by studying the basic points of endocrinology. In practice, both the experience of implementing hormonal measures while working with doctors and the study of the issue will contribute to a good understanding of this approach.

Interpreting hormone concentrations in relation to training control is different to the classic clinical evaluation. Normative values for athletes undertaking adaptive training should be first established and the results should be interpreted considering the training phase that is being undertaken. Also, because the standardization of training and diet before hormone sampling is important the involvement of a trained sport scientist is highly recommended to collect measures as well as to assist interpretation.

For future directions, the feasibility of implementing hormone measurement without further disturbing already very time-consuming training schedules is an interesting issue to address. Saliva and urine sampling are important advances that overcome some of the unpleasant characteristics of blood sampling. Nevertheless, as stated above, they are not particularly easy to implement and new non-invasive and easier to collect methods would be useful. For example, the determination of hormone levels in hair could have potential. The interest in measuring substances in hair started because of the need to detect abuse of glucocorticoids and other steroids by athletes and has recently extended to other fields, including the determination of endogenous hormone concentrations. An evident advantage of the use of hair sampling is the ease of sample collection and storage, since collection is non-invasive and hair does not decompose like other body fluids or tissues.

> The application of human scalp hair analysis to the field of psychobiology promises to be most valuable, as biological markers of stress exposure are currently covering time periods of only up to 24 h (urinary excretion rates). But there is great research interest in the effects of chronic stress over longer periods of time (e.g., several months). Therefore, the development of a reliable and valid technique to determine stress hormones in human scalp hair would fill a methodological gap.
>
> (Kirschbaum et al., 2009)

Hair strands should be carefully cut as close as possible to the scalp from a posterior vertex position. A minimum of 50 mg of hair for a 3-cm segment has to be obtained from each participant. Depending on the individual hair length, between three and nine segments are obtained from women. The most promising potential of this technique would be the creation of a retrospective calendar of endogenous cortisol exposure by hair segment analysis along the hair shaft (each hair centimetre is considered to store information about the corresponding hormone monthly concentrations). Although the technique has not been used in training contexts and its ability to produce meaningful results as a long-term biological marker has not been proved (Kirschbaum *et al.*, 2009), it is worth mentioning here for its potential to simplify hormonal information accessibility.

From a more general perspective and considering the research, the identification of valid diagnostic tools will greatly benefit from studies including larger numbers of elite athletes and observations over longer time intervals. Future investigations should focus on the causal training factors (since these are the most likely to exert control) as well as temporal changes during recovery (resting times can also be managed to a greater benefit), which may induce positive adaptations after a period of intensified training.

For the practical application of hormonal measures to training monitoring, since test results always need an individual interpretation, it is worth emphasizing the need for initial assessment of individual baseline values. Despite the cost and practical difficulties in obtaining these data, given the current state of our knowledge, the importance of information provided by basal lines should not be ignored.

Recommended reading

Resting cortisol and testosterone and testosterone to cortisol ratio

Kraemer, W. J. and Ratamess, N. A. (2005). Hormonal responses and adaptations to resistance exercise and training. *Sports Medicine*, 35, 339–361.

Urhausen, A. and Kindermann, W. (2002). Diagnosis of overtraining: what tools do we have? *Sports Medicine*, 32, 95–102.

Catecholamine excretion

Kraemer, W. J. and Ratamess, N. A. (2005). Hormonal responses and adaptations to resistance exercise and training. *Sports Medicine*, 35, 339–361.

Urhausen, A. and Kindermann, W. (2002). Diagnosis of overtraining: what tools do we have? *Sports Medicine*, 32, 95–102.

Saliva sampling

Hansen, A. M., Garde, A. H. and Persson, R. (2008). Sources of biological and methodological variation in salivary cortisol and their impact on measurement among healthy adults: a review. *Scandinavian Journal of Clinical and Laboratory Investigation*, 68, 448–458.

Kirschbaum, C. and Hellhammer, D. H. (1994). Salivary cortisol in psychoneuroendocrine research: recent developments and applications. *Psychoneuroendocrinology*, 19, 313–333.

Törnhage, C. J. (2009). Salivary cortisol for assessment of hypothalamic-pituitary-adrenal axis function. *Neuroimmunomodulation*, 16, 284–289.

Hair analyses

Gow, R., Thomson, S., Rieder, M., Van Uum, S. and Koren, G. (2010). An assessment of cortisol analysis in hair and its clinical applications. *Forensic Science International*, 196, 32–37.

Kirschbaum, C., Tietze, A., Skoluda, N. and Dettenborn, L. (2009). Hair as a retrospective calendar of cortisol production increased cortisol incorporation into hair in the third trimester of pregnancy. *Psychoneuroendocrinology*, 34, 32–37.

References

Adlercreutz, H., Härkönen, M., Kuoppasalmi, K., *et al.* (1986). Effect of training on plasma anabolic and catabolic steroid hormones and their response during physical exercise. *International Journal of Sports Medicine*, 7(Suppl. 1), 27–28.

Armstrong, L. E. and Van Heest, J. L. (2002). The unknown mechanism of the overtraining syndrome: clues from depression and psychoneuroimmunology. *Sports Medicine*, 32, 185–209.

Bompa, T. (1983). *Theory and Methodology of Training: the Key to Athletic Performance*. Dubuque, IA: Kendall/Hunt.

Bonete, E. and Suay, F. (2003). Conceptos básicos y terminología del sobreentrenamiento. [Basic concepts and terminology of overtraining]. In F. Suay (ed.), *El síndrome de sobreentrenamiento: una visión desde la psicobiología del deporte*. Barcelona: Paidotribo.

Brink, M. S., Visscher, C., Coutts, A. J. and Lemmink, K. A. P. M. (2010). Changes in perceived stress and recovery in overreached young elite soccer players. *Scandinavian Journal of Medicine and Science in Sports*, [Epub ahead of print].

Budgett, R., Newsholme, E., Lehmann, M., *et al.* (2000). Redefining the overtraining syndrome as the unexplained underperformance syndrome. *British Journal of Sports Medicine*, 34, 67–68.

Fry, R. W., Morton, A. R. and Keast, D. (1991). Overtraining in athletes: an update. *Sports Medicine*, 12, 32–65.

Gouarné, C., Groussard, C., Gratas-Delamarche, A., Delamarche, P. and Duclos, M. (2005). Overnight urinary cortisol and cortisone add new insights into adaptation to training. *Medicine and Science in Sports and Exercise*, 37, 1157–1167.

Granger, D. A. and Kivlighan, K. T. (2003). Integrating biological, behavioral, and social levels of analysis in early child development: progress, problems, and prospects. *Child Development*, 74, 1058–1063.

Hackney, A. C. and Zack, E. (2006). Physiological day-to-day variability of select hormones at rest in exercise-trained men. *Journal of Endocrinological Investigation*, 29, RC9–12.

Halson, S. L. and Jeukendrup, A. E. (2004). Does overtraining exist? An analysis of over-reaching and overtraining research. *Sports Medicine*, 34, 967–981.

Hawley, C. J. and Schoene, R. B. (2003). Overtraining syndrome: a guide to diagnosis, treatment, and prevention. *The Physician and Sportsmedicine*, 31, 25–31.

Hedelin, R., Kentta, G., Wiklund, U., Bjerle, P. and Henriksson-Larsen, K. (2000). Short-term overtraining: effects on performance, circulatory responses, and heart rate variability. *Medicine and Science in Sports and Exercise*, 32, 1480–1484.

Kellmann, M. (ed.) (2002). *Enhancing Recovery: Preventing underperformance in athletes*. Champaign, IL: Human Kinetics.

Kenttä, G., Hassmén, P. and Raglin, J. S. (2001). Training practices and overtraining syndrome in Swedish age-group athletes. *International Journal of Sports Medicine*, 22, 460–465.

Kirschbaum, C., Tietze, A., Skoluda, N. and Dettenborn, L. (2009). Hair as a retrospective calendar of cortisol production – increased cortisol incorporation into hair in the third trimester of pregnancy. *Psychoneuroendocrinology*, 34, 32–37.

Kraemer, W. J. and Ratamess, N. A. (2005). Hormonal responses and adaptations to resistance exercise and training. *Sports Medicine*, 35, 339–361.

Kreider, R., Fry, A. C. and O'Toole, M. (1998). Overtraining in sport: terms, definitions, and prevalence. In R. Kreider, A. C. Fry and M. O'Toole (eds), *Overtraining in Sport* (pp. vii–ix). Champaign, IL: Human Kinetics.

Kudielka, B. M. and Wüst, S. (2010). Human models in acute and chronic stress: assessing determinants of individual hypothalamus-pituitary-adrenal axis activity and reactivity. *Stress*, 13, 1–14.

Lac, G. and Maso, F. (2004). Biological markers for the follow-up of athletes throughout the training season. *Pathologie Biologie (Paris)*, 52, 43–49.

Lehmann, M., Schnee, W., Scheu, R., Stockhausen, W. and Bachl. N. (1992a). Decreased nocturnal catecholamine excretion: parameter for an overtraining syndrome in athletes? *International Journal of Sports Medicine*, 13, 236–242.

Lehmann, M., Baumgartl, P., Wiesenack, C., *et al.* (1992b). Training-overtraining: influence of a defined increase in training volume vs training intensity on performance, catecholamines and some metabolic parameters in experienced middle- and long-distance runners. *European Journal of Applied Physiology and Occupational Physiology*, 64, 169–177.

Lehmann, M., Foster, C. and Keul, J. (1993). Overtraining in endurance athletes: a brief review. *Medicine and Science in Sports and Exercise*, 25, 854–862.

Lehmann, M., Foster, C., Gastmann, U., Keizer, H. and Steinacker, J. (1999). Definitions, types, symptoms, findings, underlying mechanisms, and frequency of overtraining and overtraining syndrome. In M. Lehmann, C. Foster, U. Gastmann, H. Keizer and J. Steinacker (eds), *Overload, Performance Incompetence, and Regeneration in Sport* (pp. 1–6). New York: Kluwer Academic/Plenum.

Mackinnon, L. T., Hooper, S., Jones, S., Gordon, R. and Bachmann, A. (1997). Hormonal, immunological, and haematological responses to intensified training in elite swimmers. *Medicine and Science in Sports and Exercise*, 29, 1637–1645.

Matos, N. F., Winsley, R. J. and Williams, C. A. (2011). Prevalence of non-functional overreaching/overtraining in young English athletes. *Medicine and Science in Sports and Exercise*, 43, 1287–1294.

McEwen, B. and Lasley, E. N. (2003). Allostatic load: when protection gives way to damage. *Advances in Mind-Body Medicine*, 19, 28–33.

Meeusen, R., Duclos, M., Gleeson, M., Rietjens, G., Steinacker, J. and Urhausen, A. (2006). Prevention, diagnosis and treatment of the overtraining syndrome. *European Journal of Sport Science*, 6, 1–14.

Morgan, W. P., O'Connor, P. J., Sparling, P. B. and Pate, R. R. (1987). Psychological characterization of the elite female distance runner. *International Journal of Sports Medicine*, 8, 124–131.

Morgan, W. P., O'Connor, P. J., Ellickson, K. A. and Bradley, P. W. (1988). Personality structure, mood states, and performance in elite male distance runners. *International Journal of Sport Psychology*, 19, 247–263.

Peterson, K. (2005). Overtraining: balancing practice and performance. In S. Murphy (ed.). *The Sports Psychologist's Handbook* (pp. 49–70). Champaign, IL: Human Kinetics.

Purvis, D., Gonsalves, S. and Deuster, P. A. (2010). Physiological and psychological fatigue in extreme conditions: overtraining and elite athletes. *PM and R*, 2, 442–450.

Raglin, J. S., Sawamura, S., Alexiou, S., Hassmén, P. and Kenttä, G. (2000). Training practices and staleness in 13–18 year old swimmers: A cross-cultural study. *Pediatric Sports Medicine*, 12, 61–70.

Rowbottom, D. G and Green, K. J. (2000). Acute exercise effects on the immune system. *Medicine and Science in Sports and Exercise*, 32(Suppl. 7), 396–405.

Salvador, A. (2005). Coping with competitive situations in humans. *Neuroscience and Biobehavioral Reviews*, 29, 195–205.

Steinacker, J. M., Lormes, W., Reissnecker, S. and Liu, Y. (2004). New aspects of the hormone and cytokine response to training. *European Journal of Applied Physiology*, 91, 382–391.

Suay, F. and Salvador, A. (2003). Marcadores hormonales de sobreentrenamiento [Hormonal markers of overtraining]. In F. Suay (ed.), *El Síndrome de Sobreentrenamiento: una Visión desde la Psicobiología del Deporte [The Overtraining Syndrome: A vision from Sports Psychobiology]* (pp. 80–102). Barcelona: Paidotribo.

Suay, F., Sanchis, C. and Salvador, A. (1997). Marcadores hormonales del síndrome de sobre entrenamiento. [Hormonal markers of overtraining syndrome]. *Revista de Psicología del Deporte*, 11, 21–39.

Suay, F., Salvador, A. and Ricarte, J. (1998). Indicadores psicológicos de sobreentrenamiento y agotamiento. [Psychological markers of overtraining and staleness]. *Revista de Psicología del Deporte*, 13, 7–25.

Swaab, D. F., Bao, A. M. and Lucassen, P. J. (2005). The stress system in the human brain in depression and neurodegeneration. *Ageing Research Review*, 4, 141–194.

Urhausen, A. and Kindermann, W. (2002). Diagnosis of overtraining: what tools do we have? *Sports Medicine*, 32, 95–102.

Urhausen, A., Gabriel, H. and Kindermann, W. (1995). Blood hormones as markers of training stress and overtraining. *Sports Medicine*, 20, 251–276.

Urhausen, A., Gabriel, H. H. and Kindermann, W. (1998). Impaired pituitary hormonal response to exhaustive exercise in overtrained endurance athletes. *Medicine and Science in Sports and Exercise*, 30, 407–414.

Yilmaz, G., Yilmaz, F. M., Hakligör, A. and Yücel, D. (2008). Are preservatives necessary in 24-hour urine measurements? *Clinical Biochemistry*, 41, 899–901.

Index

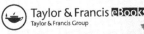 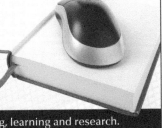